Diabetes
Log book

This book belongs to :

....

....

Date:			Day:			Mood:		
	☕ Breakfast		🍴 Lunch		✗ Dinner		🛏 Bedtime	
	Time	Level	Time	Level	Time	Level	Time	Level
Pre								
Pos								
Notes:								

Date:			Day:			Mood:		
	☕ Breakfast		🍴 Lunch		✗ Dinner		🛏 Bedtime	
	Time	Level	Time	Level	Time	Level	Time	Level
Pre								
Pos								
Notes:								

Date:			Day:			Mood:		
	☕ Breakfast		🍴 Lunch		✗ Dinner		🛏 Bedtime	
	Time	Level	Time	Level	Time	Level	Time	Level
Pre								
Pos								
Notes:								

Date:			Day:			Mood:		
	☕ Breakfast		🍴 Lunch		✗ Dinner		🛏 Bedtime	
	Time	Level	Time	Level	Time	Level	Time	Level
Pre								
Pos								
Notes:								

Date:			Day:			Mood:		
	☕ Breakfast		🍴 Lunch		✗ Dinner		🛏 Bedtime	
	Time	Level	Time	Level	Time	Level	Time	Level
Pre								
Pos								
Notes:								

Date:			Day:			Mood:		
	☕ Breakfast		🍴 Lunch		✗ Dinner		🛏 Bedtime	
	Time	Level	Time	Level	Time	Level	Time	Level
Pre								
Pos								
Notes:								

Date:			Day:			Mood:		
	☕ Breakfast		🍴 Lunch		✕ Dinner		🛏 Bedtime	
	Time	Level	Time	Level	Time	Level	Time	Level
Pre								
Pos								
Notes:								

Date:			Day:			Mood:		
	☕ Breakfast		🍴 Lunch		✕ Dinner		🛏 Bedtime	
	Time	Level	Time	Level	Time	Level	Time	Level
Pre								
Pos								
Notes:								

Date:			Day:			Mood:		
	☕ Breakfast		🍴 Lunch		✕ Dinner		🛏 Bedtime	
	Time	Level	Time	Level	Time	Level	Time	Level
Pre								
Pos								
Notes:								

Date:			Day:			Mood:		
	☕ Breakfast		🍴 Lunch		✕ Dinner		🛏 Bedtime	
	Time	Level	Time	Level	Time	Level	Time	Level
Pre								
Pos								
Notes:								

Date:			Day:			Mood:		
	☕ Breakfast		🍴 Lunch		✕ Dinner		🛏 Bedtime	
	Time	Level	Time	Level	Time	Level	Time	Level
Pre								
Pos								
Notes:								

Date:			Day:			Mood:		
	☕ Breakfast		🍴 Lunch		✕ Dinner		🛏 Bedtime	
	Time	Level	Time	Level	Time	Level	Time	Level
Pre								
Pos								
Notes:								

Date:		Day:			Mood:		
	☕ Breakfast		🍴 Lunch		✗ Dinner		🛏 Bedtime	
	Time	Level	Time	Level	Time	Level	Time	Level
Pre								
Pos								

Notes:

Date:		Day:			Mood:		
	☕ Breakfast		🍴 Lunch		✗ Dinner		🛏 Bedtime	
	Time	Level	Time	Level	Time	Level	Time	Level
Pre								
Pos								

Notes:

Date:		Day:			Mood:		
	☕ Breakfast		🍴 Lunch		✗ Dinner		🛏 Bedtime	
	Time	Level	Time	Level	Time	Level	Time	Level
Pre								
Pos								

Notes:

Date:		Day:			Mood:		
	☕ Breakfast		🍴 Lunch		✗ Dinner		🛏 Bedtime	
	Time	Level	Time	Level	Time	Level	Time	Level
Pre								
Pos								

Notes:

Date:		Day:			Mood:		
	☕ Breakfast		🍴 Lunch		✗ Dinner		🛏 Bedtime	
	Time	Level	Time	Level	Time	Level	Time	Level
Pre								
Pos								

Notes:

Date:		Day:			Mood:		
	☕ Breakfast		🍴 Lunch		✗ Dinner		🛏 Bedtime	
	Time	Level	Time	Level	Time	Level	Time	Level
Pre								
Pos								

Notes:

Date:			Day:			Mood:		
	☕ Breakfast		🍴 Lunch		✕ Dinner		🛏 Bedtime	
	Time	Level	Time	Level	Time	Level	Time	Level
Pre								
Pos								
Notes:								

Date:			Day:			Mood:		
	☕ Breakfast		🍴 Lunch		✕ Dinner		🛏 Bedtime	
	Time	Level	Time	Level	Time	Level	Time	Level
Pre								
Pos								
Notes:								

Date:			Day:			Mood:		
	☕ Breakfast		🍴 Lunch		✕ Dinner		🛏 Bedtime	
	Time	Level	Time	Level	Time	Level	Time	Level
Pre								
Pos								
Notes:								

Date:			Day:			Mood:		
	☕ Breakfast		🍴 Lunch		✕ Dinner		🛏 Bedtime	
	Time	Level	Time	Level	Time	Level	Time	Level
Pre								
Pos								
Notes:								

Date:			Day:			Mood:		
	☕ Breakfast		🍴 Lunch		✕ Dinner		🛏 Bedtime	
	Time	Level	Time	Level	Time	Level	Time	Level
Pre								
Pos								
Notes:								

Date:			Day:			Mood:		
	☕ Breakfast		🍴 Lunch		✕ Dinner		🛏 Bedtime	
	Time	Level	Time	Level	Time	Level	Time	Level
Pre								
Pos								
Notes:								

Date:			Day:			Mood:		
	☕ Breakfast		🍴 Lunch		✕ Dinner		🛏 Bedtime	
	Time	Level	Time	Level	Time	Level	Time	Level
Pre								
Pos								

Notes:

Date:			Day:			Mood:		
	☕ Breakfast		🍴 Lunch		✕ Dinner		🛏 Bedtime	
	Time	Level	Time	Level	Time	Level	Time	Level
Pre								
Pos								

Notes:

Date:			Day:			Mood:		
	☕ Breakfast		🍴 Lunch		✕ Dinner		🛏 Bedtime	
	Time	Level	Time	Level	Time	Level	Time	Level
Pre								
Pos								

Notes:

Date:			Day:			Mood:		
	☕ Breakfast		🍴 Lunch		✕ Dinner		🛏 Bedtime	
	Time	Level	Time	Level	Time	Level	Time	Level
Pre								
Pos								

Notes:

Date:			Day:			Mood:		
	☕ Breakfast		🍴 Lunch		✕ Dinner		🛏 Bedtime	
	Time	Level	Time	Level	Time	Level	Time	Level
Pre								
Pos								

Notes:

Date:			Day:			Mood:		
	☕ Breakfast		🍴 Lunch		✕ Dinner		🛏 Bedtime	
	Time	Level	Time	Level	Time	Level	Time	Level
Pre								
Pos								

Notes:

Date:			Day:			Mood:		
	☕ Breakfast		🍴 Lunch		✗ Dinner		🛏 Bedtime	
	Time	Level	Time	Level	Time	Level	Time	Level
Pre								
Pos								
Notes:								

Date:			Day:			Mood:		
	☕ Breakfast		🍴 Lunch		✗ Dinner		🛏 Bedtime	
	Time	Level	Time	Level	Time	Level	Time	Level
Pre								
Pos								
Notes:								

Date:			Day:			Mood:		
	☕ Breakfast		🍴 Lunch		✗ Dinner		🛏 Bedtime	
	Time	Level	Time	Level	Time	Level	Time	Level
Pre								
Pos								
Notes:								

Date:			Day:			Mood:		
	☕ Breakfast		🍴 Lunch		✗ Dinner		🛏 Bedtime	
	Time	Level	Time	Level	Time	Level	Time	Level
Pre								
Pos								
Notes:								

Date:			Day:			Mood:		
	☕ Breakfast		🍴 Lunch		✗ Dinner		🛏 Bedtime	
	Time	Level	Time	Level	Time	Level	Time	Level
Pre								
Pos								
Notes:								

Date:			Day:			Mood:		
	☕ Breakfast		🍴 Lunch		✗ Dinner		🛏 Bedtime	
	Time	Level	Time	Level	Time	Level	Time	Level
Pre								
Pos								
Notes:								

Date:			Day:				Mood:		
	☕ Breakfast		🍴 Lunch		✕ Dinner		🛏 Bedtime		
	Time	Level	Time	Level	Time	Level	Time	Level
Pre								
Pos								

Notes:

Date:			Day:				Mood:		
	☕ Breakfast		🍴 Lunch		✕ Dinner		🛏 Bedtime		
	Time	Level	Time	Level	Time	Level	Time	Level
Pre								
Pos								

Notes:

Date:			Day:				Mood:		
	☕ Breakfast		🍴 Lunch		✕ Dinner		🛏 Bedtime		
	Time	Level	Time	Level	Time	Level	Time	Level
Pre								
Pos								

Notes:

Date:			Day:				Mood:		
	☕ Breakfast		🍴 Lunch		✕ Dinner		🛏 Bedtime		
	Time	Level	Time	Level	Time	Level	Time	Level
Pre								
Pos								

Notes:

Date:			Day:				Mood:		
	☕ Breakfast		🍴 Lunch		✕ Dinner		🛏 Bedtime		
	Time	Level	Time	Level	Time	Level	Time	Level
Pre								
Pos								

Notes:

Date:			Day:				Mood:		
	☕ Breakfast		🍴 Lunch		✕ Dinner		🛏 Bedtime		
	Time	Level	Time	Level	Time	Level	Time	Level
Pre								
Pos								

Notes:

Date:				Day:			Mood:		
	☕ Breakfast		🍴 Lunch		✗ Dinner		🛏 Bedtime		
	Time	Level	Time	Level	Time	Level	Time	Level	
Pre									
Pos									
Notes:									

Date:				Day:			Mood:		
	☕ Breakfast		🍴 Lunch		✗ Dinner		🛏 Bedtime		
	Time	Level	Time	Level	Time	Level	Time	Level	
Pre									
Pos									
Notes:									

Date:				Day:			Mood:		
	☕ Breakfast		🍴 Lunch		✗ Dinner		🛏 Bedtime		
	Time	Level	Time	Level	Time	Level	Time	Level	
Pre									
Pos									
Notes:									

Date:				Day:			Mood:		
	☕ Breakfast		🍴 Lunch		✗ Dinner		🛏 Bedtime		
	Time	Level	Time	Level	Time	Level	Time	Level	
Pre									
Pos									
Notes:									

Date:				Day:			Mood:		
	☕ Breakfast		🍴 Lunch		✗ Dinner		🛏 Bedtime		
	Time	Level	Time	Level	Time	Level	Time	Level	
Pre									
Pos									
Notes:									

Date:				Day:			Mood:		
	☕ Breakfast		🍴 Lunch		✗ Dinner		🛏 Bedtime		
	Time	Level	Time	Level	Time	Level	Time	Level	
Pre									
Pos									
Notes:									

Date:			Day:			Mood:		
	☕ Breakfast		🍲 Lunch		✕ Dinner		🛏 Bedtime	
	Time	Level	Time	Level	Time	Level	Time	Level
Pre								
Pos								

Notes:

Date:			Day:			Mood:		
	☕ Breakfast		🍲 Lunch		✕ Dinner		🛏 Bedtime	
	Time	Level	Time	Level	Time	Level	Time	Level
Pre								
Pos								

Notes:

Date:			Day:			Mood:		
	☕ Breakfast		🍲 Lunch		✕ Dinner		🛏 Bedtime	
	Time	Level	Time	Level	Time	Level	Time	Level
Pre								
Pos								

Notes:

Date:			Day:			Mood:		
	☕ Breakfast		🍲 Lunch		✕ Dinner		🛏 Bedtime	
	Time	Level	Time	Level	Time	Level	Time	Level
Pre								
Pos								

Notes:

Date:			Day:			Mood:		
	☕ Breakfast		🍲 Lunch		✕ Dinner		🛏 Bedtime	
	Time	Level	Time	Level	Time	Level	Time	Level
Pre								
Pos								

Notes:

Date:			Day:			Mood:		
	☕ Breakfast		🍲 Lunch		✕ Dinner		🛏 Bedtime	
	Time	Level	Time	Level	Time	Level	Time	Level
Pre								
Pos								

Notes:

Date:			Day:			Mood:		
	☕ Breakfast		🍴 Lunch		✗ Dinner		🛏 Bedtime	
	Time	Level	Time	Level	Time	Level	Time	Level
Pre								
Pos								
Notes:								

Date:			Day:			Mood:		
	☕ Breakfast		🍴 Lunch		✗ Dinner		🛏 Bedtime	
	Time	Level	Time	Level	Time	Level	Time	Level
Pre								
Pos								
Notes:								

Date:			Day:			Mood:		
	☕ Breakfast		🍴 Lunch		✗ Dinner		🛏 Bedtime	
	Time	Level	Time	Level	Time	Level	Time	Level
Pre								
Pos								
Notes:								

Date:			Day:			Mood:		
	☕ Breakfast		🍴 Lunch		✗ Dinner		🛏 Bedtime	
	Time	Level	Time	Level	Time	Level	Time	Level
Pre								
Pos								
Notes:								

Date:			Day:			Mood:		
	☕ Breakfast		🍴 Lunch		✗ Dinner		🛏 Bedtime	
	Time	Level	Time	Level	Time	Level	Time	Level
Pre								
Pos								
Notes:								

Date:			Day:			Mood:		
	☕ Breakfast		🍴 Lunch		✗ Dinner		🛏 Bedtime	
	Time	Level	Time	Level	Time	Level	Time	Level
Pre								
Pos								
Notes:								

Date:			Day:			Mood:		
	☕ Breakfast		🍴 Lunch		✗ Dinner		🛏 Bedtime	
	Time	Level	Time	Level	Time	Level	Time	Level
Pre								
Pos								
Notes:								

Date:			Day:			Mood:		
	☕ Breakfast		🍴 Lunch		✗ Dinner		🛏 Bedtime	
	Time	Level	Time	Level	Time	Level	Time	Level
Pre								
Pos								
Notes:								

Date:			Day:			Mood:		
	☕ Breakfast		🍴 Lunch		✗ Dinner		🛏 Bedtime	
	Time	Level	Time	Level	Time	Level	Time	Level
Pre								
Pos								
Notes:								

Date:			Day:			Mood:		
	☕ Breakfast		🍴 Lunch		✗ Dinner		🛏 Bedtime	
	Time	Level	Time	Level	Time	Level	Time	Level
Pre								
Pos								
Notes:								

Date:			Day:			Mood:		
	☕ Breakfast		🍴 Lunch		✗ Dinner		🛏 Bedtime	
	Time	Level	Time	Level	Time	Level	Time	Level
Pre								
Pos								
Notes:								

Date:			Day:			Mood:		
	☕ Breakfast		🍴 Lunch		✗ Dinner		🛏 Bedtime	
	Time	Level	Time	Level	Time	Level	Time	Level
Pre								
Pos								
Notes:								

Date:		Day:		Mood:	

	☕ Breakfast		🍽 Lunch		✗ Dinner		🛏 Bedtime	
	Time	Level	Time	Level	Time	Level	Time	Level
Pre								
Pos								

Notes:

Date:		Day:		Mood:	

	☕ Breakfast		🍽 Lunch		✗ Dinner		🛏 Bedtime	
	Time	Level	Time	Level	Time	Level	Time	Level
Pre								
Pos								

Notes:

Date:		Day:		Mood:	

	☕ Breakfast		🍽 Lunch		✗ Dinner		🛏 Bedtime	
	Time	Level	Time	Level	Time	Level	Time	Level
Pre								
Pos								

Notes:

Date:		Day:		Mood:	

	☕ Breakfast		🍽 Lunch		✗ Dinner		🛏 Bedtime	
	Time	Level	Time	Level	Time	Level	Time	Level
Pre								
Pos								

Notes:

Date:		Day:		Mood:	

	☕ Breakfast		🍽 Lunch		✗ Dinner		🛏 Bedtime	
	Time	Level	Time	Level	Time	Level	Time	Level
Pre								
Pos								

Notes:

Date:		Day:		Mood:	

	☕ Breakfast		🍽 Lunch		✗ Dinner		🛏 Bedtime	
	Time	Level	Time	Level	Time	Level	Time	Level
Pre								
Pos								

Notes:

Date:			Day:			Mood:		
	☕ Breakfast		🍴 Lunch		✕ Dinner		🛏 Bedtime	
	Time	Level	Time	Level	Time	Level	Time	Level
Pre								
Pos								

Notes:

Date:			Day:			Mood:		
	☕ Breakfast		🍴 Lunch		✕ Dinner		🛏 Bedtime	
	Time	Level	Time	Level	Time	Level	Time	Level
Pre								
Pos								

Notes:

Date:			Day:			Mood:		
	☕ Breakfast		🍴 Lunch		✕ Dinner		🛏 Bedtime	
	Time	Level	Time	Level	Time	Level	Time	Level
Pre								
Pos								

Notes:

Date:			Day:			Mood:		
	☕ Breakfast		🍴 Lunch		✕ Dinner		🛏 Bedtime	
	Time	Level	Time	Level	Time	Level	Time	Level
Pre								
Pos								

Notes:

Date:			Day:			Mood:		
	☕ Breakfast		🍴 Lunch		✕ Dinner		🛏 Bedtime	
	Time	Level	Time	Level	Time	Level	Time	Level
Pre								
Pos								

Notes:

Date:			Day:			Mood:		
	☕ Breakfast		🍴 Lunch		✕ Dinner		🛏 Bedtime	
	Time	Level	Time	Level	Time	Level	Time	Level
Pre								
Pos								

Notes:

Date:		Day:			Mood:		
	☕ Breakfast		🍴 Lunch		✕ Dinner		🛏 Bedtime
	Time	Level	Time	Level	Time	Level	Time	Level
Pre								
Pos								
Notes:								

Date:		Day:			Mood:		
	☕ Breakfast		🍴 Lunch		✕ Dinner		🛏 Bedtime
	Time	Level	Time	Level	Time	Level	Time	Level
Pre								
Pos								
Notes:								

Date:		Day:			Mood:		
	☕ Breakfast		🍴 Lunch		✕ Dinner		🛏 Bedtime
	Time	Level	Time	Level	Time	Level	Time	Level
Pre								
Pos								
Notes:								

Date:		Day:			Mood:		
	☕ Breakfast		🍴 Lunch		✕ Dinner		🛏 Bedtime
	Time	Level	Time	Level	Time	Level	Time	Level
Pre								
Pos								
Notes:								

Date:		Day:			Mood:		
	☕ Breakfast		🍴 Lunch		✕ Dinner		🛏 Bedtime
	Time	Level	Time	Level	Time	Level	Time	Level
Pre								
Pos								
Notes:								

Date:		Day:			Mood:		
	☕ Breakfast		🍴 Lunch		✕ Dinner		🛏 Bedtime
	Time	Level	Time	Level	Time	Level	Time	Level
Pre								
Pos								
Notes:								

Date:			Day:			Mood:		
	☕ Breakfast		🍴 Lunch		✗ Dinner		🛏 Bedtime	
	Time	Level	Time	Level	Time	Level	Time	Level
Pre								
Pos								
Notes:								

Date:			Day:			Mood:		
	☕ Breakfast		🍴 Lunch		✗ Dinner		🛏 Bedtime	
	Time	Level	Time	Level	Time	Level	Time	Level
Pre								
Pos								
Notes:								

Date:			Day:			Mood:		
	☕ Breakfast		🍴 Lunch		✗ Dinner		🛏 Bedtime	
	Time	Level	Time	Level	Time	Level	Time	Level
Pre								
Pos								
Notes:								

Date:			Day:			Mood:		
	☕ Breakfast		🍴 Lunch		✗ Dinner		🛏 Bedtime	
	Time	Level	Time	Level	Time	Level	Time	Level
Pre								
Pos								
Notes:								

Date:			Day:			Mood:		
	☕ Breakfast		🍴 Lunch		✗ Dinner		🛏 Bedtime	
	Time	Level	Time	Level	Time	Level	Time	Level
Pre								
Pos								
Notes:								

Date:			Day:			Mood:		
	☕ Breakfast		🍴 Lunch		✗ Dinner		🛏 Bedtime	
	Time	Level	Time	Level	Time	Level	Time	Level
Pre								
Pos								
Notes:								

Date:			Day:			Mood:		
	☕ Breakfast		🍴 Lunch		✗ Dinner		🛏 Bedtime	
	Time	Level	Time	Level	Time	Level	Time	Level
Pre								
Pos								
Notes:								

Date:			Day:			Mood:		
	☕ Breakfast		🍴 Lunch		✗ Dinner		🛏 Bedtime	
	Time	Level	Time	Level	Time	Level	Time	Level
Pre								
Pos								
Notes:								

Date:			Day:			Mood:		
	☕ Breakfast		🍴 Lunch		✗ Dinner		🛏 Bedtime	
	Time	Level	Time	Level	Time	Level	Time	Level
Pre								
Pos								
Notes:								

Date:			Day:			Mood:		
	☕ Breakfast		🍴 Lunch		✗ Dinner		🛏 Bedtime	
	Time	Level	Time	Level	Time	Level	Time	Level
Pre								
Pos								
Notes:								

Date:			Day:			Mood:		
	☕ Breakfast		🍴 Lunch		✗ Dinner		🛏 Bedtime	
	Time	Level	Time	Level	Time	Level	Time	Level
Pre								
Pos								
Notes:								

Date:			Day:			Mood:		
	☕ Breakfast		🍴 Lunch		✗ Dinner		🛏 Bedtime	
	Time	Level	Time	Level	Time	Level	Time	Level
Pre								
Pos								
Notes:								

Date:			Day:			Mood:		
	☕ Breakfast		🍔 Lunch		✗ Dinner		🛏 Bedtime	
	Time	Level	Time	Level	Time	Level	Time	Level
Pre								
Pos								
Notes:								

Date:			Day:			Mood:		
	☕ Breakfast		🍔 Lunch		✗ Dinner		🛏 Bedtime	
	Time	Level	Time	Level	Time	Level	Time	Level
Pre								
Pos								
Notes:								

Date:			Day:			Mood:		
	☕ Breakfast		🍔 Lunch		✗ Dinner		🛏 Bedtime	
	Time	Level	Time	Level	Time	Level	Time	Level
Pre								
Pos								
Notes:								

Date:			Day:			Mood:		
	☕ Breakfast		🍔 Lunch		✗ Dinner		🛏 Bedtime	
	Time	Level	Time	Level	Time	Level	Time	Level
Pre								
Pos								
Notes:								

Date:			Day:			Mood:		
	☕ Breakfast		🍔 Lunch		✗ Dinner		🛏 Bedtime	
	Time	Level	Time	Level	Time	Level	Time	Level
Pre								
Pos								
Notes:								

Date:			Day:			Mood:		
	☕ Breakfast		🍔 Lunch		✗ Dinner		🛏 Bedtime	
	Time	Level	Time	Level	Time	Level	Time	Level
Pre								
Pos								
Notes:								

Date:			Day:			Mood:		
	☕ Breakfast		🍽 Lunch		✕ Dinner		🛏 Bedtime	
	Time	Level	Time	Level	Time	Level	Time	Level
Pre								
Pos								

Notes:

Date:			Day:			Mood:		
	☕ Breakfast		🍽 Lunch		✕ Dinner		🛏 Bedtime	
	Time	Level	Time	Level	Time	Level	Time	Level
Pre								
Pos								

Notes:

Date:			Day:			Mood:		
	☕ Breakfast		🍽 Lunch		✕ Dinner		🛏 Bedtime	
	Time	Level	Time	Level	Time	Level	Time	Level
Pre								
Pos								

Notes:

Date:			Day:			Mood:		
	☕ Breakfast		🍽 Lunch		✕ Dinner		🛏 Bedtime	
	Time	Level	Time	Level	Time	Level	Time	Level
Pre								
Pos								

Notes:

Date:			Day:			Mood:		
	☕ Breakfast		🍽 Lunch		✕ Dinner		🛏 Bedtime	
	Time	Level	Time	Level	Time	Level	Time	Level
Pre								
Pos								

Notes:

Date:			Day:			Mood:		
	☕ Breakfast		🍽 Lunch		✕ Dinner		🛏 Bedtime	
	Time	Level	Time	Level	Time	Level	Time	Level
Pre								
Pos								

Notes:

Date:			Day:			Mood:		
	☕ Breakfast		🍜 Lunch		✗ Dinner		🛏 Bedtime	
	Time	Level	Time	Level	Time	Level	Time	Level
Pre								
Pos								

Notes:

Date:			Day:			Mood:		
	☕ Breakfast		🍜 Lunch		✗ Dinner		🛏 Bedtime	
	Time	Level	Time	Level	Time	Level	Time	Level
Pre								
Pos								

Notes:

Date:			Day:			Mood:		
	☕ Breakfast		🍜 Lunch		✗ Dinner		🛏 Bedtime	
	Time	Level	Time	Level	Time	Level	Time	Level
Pre								
Pos								

Notes:

Date:			Day:			Mood:		
	☕ Breakfast		🍜 Lunch		✗ Dinner		🛏 Bedtime	
	Time	Level	Time	Level	Time	Level	Time	Level
Pre								
Pos								

Notes:

Date:			Day:			Mood:		
	☕ Breakfast		🍜 Lunch		✗ Dinner		🛏 Bedtime	
	Time	Level	Time	Level	Time	Level	Time	Level
Pre								
Pos								

Notes:

Date:			Day:			Mood:		
	☕ Breakfast		🍜 Lunch		✗ Dinner		🛏 Bedtime	
	Time	Level	Time	Level	Time	Level	Time	Level
Pre								
Pos								

Notes:

Date:			Day:			Mood:		
	☕ Breakfast		🍲 Lunch		✕ Dinner		🛏 Bedtime	
	Time	Level	Time	Level	Time	Level	Time	Level
Pre								
Pos								
Notes:								

Date:			Day:			Mood:		
	☕ Breakfast		🍲 Lunch		✕ Dinner		🛏 Bedtime	
	Time	Level	Time	Level	Time	Level	Time	Level
Pre								
Pos								
Notes:								

Date:			Day:			Mood:		
	☕ Breakfast		🍲 Lunch		✕ Dinner		🛏 Bedtime	
	Time	Level	Time	Level	Time	Level	Time	Level
Pre								
Pos								
Notes:								

Date:			Day:			Mood:		
	☕ Breakfast		🍲 Lunch		✕ Dinner		🛏 Bedtime	
	Time	Level	Time	Level	Time	Level	Time	Level
Pre								
Pos								
Notes:								

Date:			Day:			Mood:		
	☕ Breakfast		🍲 Lunch		✕ Dinner		🛏 Bedtime	
	Time	Level	Time	Level	Time	Level	Time	Level
Pre								
Pos								
Notes:								

Date:			Day:			Mood:		
	☕ Breakfast		🍲 Lunch		✕ Dinner		🛏 Bedtime	
	Time	Level	Time	Level	Time	Level	Time	Level
Pre								
Pos								
Notes:								

Date:			Day:			Mood:		
	☕ Breakfast		🍴 Lunch		✗ Dinner		🛏 Bedtime	
	Time	Level	Time	Level	Time	Level	Time	Level
Pre								
Pos								

Notes:

Date:			Day:			Mood:		
	☕ Breakfast		🍴 Lunch		✗ Dinner		🛏 Bedtime	
	Time	Level	Time	Level	Time	Level	Time	Level
Pre								
Pos								

Notes:

Date:			Day:			Mood:		
	☕ Breakfast		🍴 Lunch		✗ Dinner		🛏 Bedtime	
	Time	Level	Time	Level	Time	Level	Time	Level
Pre								
Pos								

Notes:

Date:			Day:			Mood:		
	☕ Breakfast		🍴 Lunch		✗ Dinner		🛏 Bedtime	
	Time	Level	Time	Level	Time	Level	Time	Level
Pre								
Pos								

Notes:

Date:			Day:			Mood:		
	☕ Breakfast		🍴 Lunch		✗ Dinner		🛏 Bedtime	
	Time	Level	Time	Level	Time	Level	Time	Level
Pre								
Pos								

Notes:

Date:			Day:			Mood:		
	☕ Breakfast		🍴 Lunch		✗ Dinner		🛏 Bedtime	
	Time	Level	Time	Level	Time	Level	Time	Level
Pre								
Pos								

Notes:

Date:			Day:			Mood:		
	Breakfast		Lunch		Dinner		Bedtime	
	Time	Level	Time	Level	Time	Level	Time	Level
Pre								
Pos								
Notes:								

Date:			Day:			Mood:		
	Breakfast		Lunch		Dinner		Bedtime	
	Time	Level	Time	Level	Time	Level	Time	Level
Pre								
Pos								
Notes:								

Date:			Day:			Mood:		
	Breakfast		Lunch		Dinner		Bedtime	
	Time	Level	Time	Level	Time	Level	Time	Level
Pre								
Pos								
Notes:								

Date:			Day:			Mood:		
	Breakfast		Lunch		Dinner		Bedtime	
	Time	Level	Time	Level	Time	Level	Time	Level
Pre								
Pos								
Notes:								

Date:			Day:			Mood:		
	Breakfast		Lunch		Dinner		Bedtime	
	Time	Level	Time	Level	Time	Level	Time	Level
Pre								
Pos								
Notes:								

Date:			Day:			Mood:		
	Breakfast		Lunch		Dinner		Bedtime	
	Time	Level	Time	Level	Time	Level	Time	Level
Pre								
Pos								
Notes:								

Date:			Day:			Mood:		
	🍵 Breakfast		🍲 Lunch		✕ Dinner		🛏 Bedtime	
	Time	Level	Time	Level	Time	Level	Time	Level
Pre								
Pos								

Notes:

Date:			Day:			Mood:		
	🍵 Breakfast		🍲 Lunch		✕ Dinner		🛏 Bedtime	
	Time	Level	Time	Level	Time	Level	Time	Level
Pre								
Pos								

Notes:

Date:			Day:			Mood:		
	🍵 Breakfast		🍲 Lunch		✕ Dinner		🛏 Bedtime	
	Time	Level	Time	Level	Time	Level	Time	Level
Pre								
Pos								

Notes:

Date:			Day:			Mood:		
	🍵 Breakfast		🍲 Lunch		✕ Dinner		🛏 Bedtime	
	Time	Level	Time	Level	Time	Level	Time	Level
Pre								
Pos								

Notes:

Date:			Day:			Mood:		
	🍵 Breakfast		🍲 Lunch		✕ Dinner		🛏 Bedtime	
	Time	Level	Time	Level	Time	Level	Time	Level
Pre								
Pos								

Notes:

Date:			Day:			Mood:		
	🍵 Breakfast		🍲 Lunch		✕ Dinner		🛏 Bedtime	
	Time	Level	Time	Level	Time	Level	Time	Level
Pre								
Pos								

Notes:

Date:			Day:			Mood:		
	☕ Breakfast		🍴 Lunch		✗ Dinner		🛏 Bedtime	
	Time	Level	Time	Level	Time	Level	Time	Level
Pre								
Pos								

Notes:

Date:			Day:			Mood:		
	☕ Breakfast		🍴 Lunch		✗ Dinner		🛏 Bedtime	
	Time	Level	Time	Level	Time	Level	Time	Level
Pre								
Pos								

Notes:

Date:			Day:			Mood:		
	☕ Breakfast		🍴 Lunch		✗ Dinner		🛏 Bedtime	
	Time	Level	Time	Level	Time	Level	Time	Level
Pre								
Pos								

Notes:

Date:			Day:			Mood:		
	☕ Breakfast		🍴 Lunch		✗ Dinner		🛏 Bedtime	
	Time	Level	Time	Level	Time	Level	Time	Level
Pre								
Pos								

Notes:

Date:			Day:			Mood:		
	☕ Breakfast		🍴 Lunch		✗ Dinner		🛏 Bedtime	
	Time	Level	Time	Level	Time	Level	Time	Level
Pre								
Pos								

Notes:

Date:			Day:			Mood:		
	☕ Breakfast		🍴 Lunch		✗ Dinner		🛏 Bedtime	
	Time	Level	Time	Level	Time	Level	Time	Level
Pre								
Pos								

Notes:

Date:			Day:			Mood:		
	☕ Breakfast		🍲 Lunch		✕ Dinner		🛏 Bedtime	
	Time	Level	Time	Level	Time	Level	Time	Level
Pre								
Pos								

Notes:

Date:			Day:			Mood:		
	☕ Breakfast		🍲 Lunch		✕ Dinner		🛏 Bedtime	
	Time	Level	Time	Level	Time	Level	Time	Level
Pre								
Pos								

Notes:

Date:			Day:			Mood:		
	☕ Breakfast		🍲 Lunch		✕ Dinner		🛏 Bedtime	
	Time	Level	Time	Level	Time	Level	Time	Level
Pre								
Pos								

Notes:

Date:			Day:			Mood:		
	☕ Breakfast		🍲 Lunch		✕ Dinner		🛏 Bedtime	
	Time	Level	Time	Level	Time	Level	Time	Level
Pre								
Pos								

Notes:

Date:			Day:			Mood:		
	☕ Breakfast		🍲 Lunch		✕ Dinner		🛏 Bedtime	
	Time	Level	Time	Level	Time	Level	Time	Level
Pre								
Pos								

Notes:

Date:			Day:			Mood:		
	☕ Breakfast		🍲 Lunch		✕ Dinner		🛏 Bedtime	
	Time	Level	Time	Level	Time	Level	Time	Level
Pre								
Pos								

Notes:

Date:			Day:			Mood:			
	☕ Breakfast		🍔 Lunch		✗ Dinner		🛏 Bedtime		
	Time	Level	Time	Level	Time	Level	Time	Level
Pre								
Pos								
Notes:									

Date:			Day:			Mood:			
	☕ Breakfast		🍔 Lunch		✗ Dinner		🛏 Bedtime		
	Time	Level	Time	Level	Time	Level	Time	Level
Pre								
Pos								
Notes:									

Date:			Day:			Mood:			
	☕ Breakfast		🍔 Lunch		✗ Dinner		🛏 Bedtime		
	Time	Level	Time	Level	Time	Level	Time	Level
Pre								
Pos								
Notes:									

Date:			Day:			Mood:			
	☕ Breakfast		🍔 Lunch		✗ Dinner		🛏 Bedtime		
	Time	Level	Time	Level	Time	Level	Time	Level
Pre								
Pos								
Notes:									

Date:			Day:			Mood:			
	☕ Breakfast		🍔 Lunch		✗ Dinner		🛏 Bedtime		
	Time	Level	Time	Level	Time	Level	Time	Level
Pre								
Pos								
Notes:									

Date:			Day:			Mood:			
	☕ Breakfast		🍔 Lunch		✗ Dinner		🛏 Bedtime		
	Time	Level	Time	Level	Time	Level	Time	Level
Pre								
Pos								
Notes:									

Date:		Day:			Mood:		
	🍵 Breakfast		🍴 Lunch		✗ Dinner		🛏 Bedtime
	Time	Level	Time	Level	Time	Level	Time	Level
Pre								
Pos								

Notes:

Date:		Day:			Mood:		
	🍵 Breakfast		🍴 Lunch		✗ Dinner		🛏 Bedtime
	Time	Level	Time	Level	Time	Level	Time	Level
Pre								
Pos								

Notes:

Date:		Day:			Mood:		
	🍵 Breakfast		🍴 Lunch		✗ Dinner		🛏 Bedtime
	Time	Level	Time	Level	Time	Level	Time	Level
Pre								
Pos								

Notes:

Date:		Day:			Mood:		
	🍵 Breakfast		🍴 Lunch		✗ Dinner		🛏 Bedtime
	Time	Level	Time	Level	Time	Level	Time	Level
Pre								
Pos								

Notes:

Date:		Day:			Mood:		
	🍵 Breakfast		🍴 Lunch		✗ Dinner		🛏 Bedtime
	Time	Level	Time	Level	Time	Level	Time	Level
Pre								
Pos								

Notes:

Date:		Day:			Mood:		
	🍵 Breakfast		🍴 Lunch		✗ Dinner		🛏 Bedtime
	Time	Level	Time	Level	Time	Level	Time	Level
Pre								
Pos								

Notes:

| Date: | | Day: | | Mood: | |

	Breakfast		Lunch		Dinner		Bedtime	
	Time	Level	Time	Level	Time	Level	Time	Level
Pre								
Pos								

Notes:

| Date: | | Day: | | Mood: | |

	Breakfast		Lunch		Dinner		Bedtime	
	Time	Level	Time	Level	Time	Level	Time	Level
Pre								
Pos								

Notes:

| Date: | | Day: | | Mood: | |

	Breakfast		Lunch		Dinner		Bedtime	
	Time	Level	Time	Level	Time	Level	Time	Level
Pre								
Pos								

Notes:

| Date: | | Day: | | Mood: | |

	Breakfast		Lunch		Dinner		Bedtime	
	Time	Level	Time	Level	Time	Level	Time	Level
Pre								
Pos								

Notes:

| Date: | | Day: | | Mood: | |

	Breakfast		Lunch		Dinner		Bedtime	
	Time	Level	Time	Level	Time	Level	Time	Level
Pre								
Pos								

Notes:

| Date: | | Day: | | Mood: | |

	Breakfast		Lunch		Dinner		Bedtime	
	Time	Level	Time	Level	Time	Level	Time	Level
Pre								
Pos								

Notes:

Date:			Day:			Mood:		
	☕ Breakfast		🍝 Lunch		✗ Dinner		🛏 Bedtime	
	Time	Level	Time	Level	Time	Level	Time	Level
Pre								
Pos								

Notes:

Date:			Day:			Mood:		
	☕ Breakfast		🍝 Lunch		✗ Dinner		🛏 Bedtime	
	Time	Level	Time	Level	Time	Level	Time	Level
Pre								
Pos								

Notes:

Date:			Day:			Mood:		
	☕ Breakfast		🍝 Lunch		✗ Dinner		🛏 Bedtime	
	Time	Level	Time	Level	Time	Level	Time	Level
Pre								
Pos								

Notes:

Date:			Day:			Mood:		
	☕ Breakfast		🍝 Lunch		✗ Dinner		🛏 Bedtime	
	Time	Level	Time	Level	Time	Level	Time	Level
Pre								
Pos								

Notes:

Date:			Day:			Mood:		
	☕ Breakfast		🍝 Lunch		✗ Dinner		🛏 Bedtime	
	Time	Level	Time	Level	Time	Level	Time	Level
Pre								
Pos								

Notes:

Date:			Day:			Mood:		
	☕ Breakfast		🍝 Lunch		✗ Dinner		🛏 Bedtime	
	Time	Level	Time	Level	Time	Level	Time	Level
Pre								
Pos								

Notes:

Date:			Day:			Mood:			
	☕ Breakfast		🍔 Lunch		✗ Dinner		🛏 Bedtime		
	Time	Level	Time	Level	Time	Level	Time	Level
Pre								
Pos								
Notes:								

Date:			Day:			Mood:			
	☕ Breakfast		🍔 Lunch		✗ Dinner		🛏 Bedtime		
	Time	Level	Time	Level	Time	Level	Time	Level
Pre								
Pos								
Notes:								

Date:			Day:			Mood:			
	☕ Breakfast		🍔 Lunch		✗ Dinner		🛏 Bedtime		
	Time	Level	Time	Level	Time	Level	Time	Level
Pre								
Pos								
Notes:								

Date:			Day:			Mood:			
	☕ Breakfast		🍔 Lunch		✗ Dinner		🛏 Bedtime		
	Time	Level	Time	Level	Time	Level	Time	Level
Pre								
Pos								
Notes:								

Date:			Day:			Mood:			
	☕ Breakfast		🍔 Lunch		✗ Dinner		🛏 Bedtime		
	Time	Level	Time	Level	Time	Level	Time	Level
Pre								
Pos								
Notes:								

Date:			Day:			Mood:			
	☕ Breakfast		🍔 Lunch		✗ Dinner		🛏 Bedtime		
	Time	Level	Time	Level	Time	Level	Time	Level
Pre								
Pos								
Notes:								

Date:			Day:			Mood:			
	☕ Breakfast		🍴 Lunch		✗ Dinner		🛏 Bedtime		
	Time	Level	Time	Level	Time	Level	Time	Level
Pre								
Pos								
Notes:									

Date:			Day:			Mood:			
	☕ Breakfast		🍴 Lunch		✗ Dinner		🛏 Bedtime		
	Time	Level	Time	Level	Time	Level	Time	Level
Pre								
Pos								
Notes:									

Date:			Day:			Mood:			
	☕ Breakfast		🍴 Lunch		✗ Dinner		🛏 Bedtime		
	Time	Level	Time	Level	Time	Level	Time	Level
Pre								
Pos								
Notes:									

Date:			Day:			Mood:			
	☕ Breakfast		🍴 Lunch		✗ Dinner		🛏 Bedtime		
	Time	Level	Time	Level	Time	Level	Time	Level
Pre								
Pos								
Notes:									

Date:			Day:			Mood:			
	☕ Breakfast		🍴 Lunch		✗ Dinner		🛏 Bedtime		
	Time	Level	Time	Level	Time	Level	Time	Level
Pre								
Pos								
Notes:									

Date:			Day:			Mood:			
	☕ Breakfast		🍴 Lunch		✗ Dinner		🛏 Bedtime		
	Time	Level	Time	Level	Time	Level	Time	Level
Pre								
Pos								
Notes:									

Date:			Day:			Mood:		
	☕ Breakfast		🍴 Lunch		✗ Dinner		🛏 Bedtime	
	Time	Level	Time	Level	Time	Level	Time	Level
Pre								
Pos								
Notes:								

Date:			Day:			Mood:		
	☕ Breakfast		🍴 Lunch		✗ Dinner		🛏 Bedtime	
	Time	Level	Time	Level	Time	Level	Time	Level
Pre								
Pos								
Notes:								

Date:			Day:			Mood:		
	☕ Breakfast		🍴 Lunch		✗ Dinner		🛏 Bedtime	
	Time	Level	Time	Level	Time	Level	Time	Level
Pre								
Pos								
Notes:								

Date:			Day:			Mood:		
	☕ Breakfast		🍴 Lunch		✗ Dinner		🛏 Bedtime	
	Time	Level	Time	Level	Time	Level	Time	Level
Pre								
Pos								
Notes:								

Date:			Day:			Mood:		
	☕ Breakfast		🍴 Lunch		✗ Dinner		🛏 Bedtime	
	Time	Level	Time	Level	Time	Level	Time	Level
Pre								
Pos								
Notes:								

Date:			Day:			Mood:		
	☕ Breakfast		🍴 Lunch		✗ Dinner		🛏 Bedtime	
	Time	Level	Time	Level	Time	Level	Time	Level
Pre								
Pos								
Notes:								

Date:			Day:			Mood:		
	☕ Breakfast		🍽 Lunch		✕ Dinner		🛏 Bedtime	
	Time	Level	Time	Level	Time	Level	Time	Level
Pre								
Pos								

Notes:

Date:			Day:			Mood:		
	☕ Breakfast		🍽 Lunch		✕ Dinner		🛏 Bedtime	
	Time	Level	Time	Level	Time	Level	Time	Level
Pre								
Pos								

Notes:

Date:			Day:			Mood:		
	☕ Breakfast		🍽 Lunch		✕ Dinner		🛏 Bedtime	
	Time	Level	Time	Level	Time	Level	Time	Level
Pre								
Pos								

Notes:

Date:			Day:			Mood:		
	☕ Breakfast		🍽 Lunch		✕ Dinner		🛏 Bedtime	
	Time	Level	Time	Level	Time	Level	Time	Level
Pre								
Pos								

Notes:

Date:			Day:			Mood:		
	☕ Breakfast		🍽 Lunch		✕ Dinner		🛏 Bedtime	
	Time	Level	Time	Level	Time	Level	Time	Level
Pre								
Pos								

Notes:

Date:			Day:			Mood:		
	☕ Breakfast		🍽 Lunch		✕ Dinner		🛏 Bedtime	
	Time	Level	Time	Level	Time	Level	Time	Level
Pre								
Pos								

Notes:

Date:		Day:			Mood:		
	☕ Breakfast		🍔 Lunch		✗ Dinner		🛏 Bedtime
	Time	Level	Time	Level	Time	Level	Time	Level
Pre								
Pos								

Notes:

Date:		Day:			Mood:		
	☕ Breakfast		🍔 Lunch		✗ Dinner		🛏 Bedtime
	Time	Level	Time	Level	Time	Level	Time	Level
Pre								
Pos								

Notes:

Date:		Day:			Mood:		
	☕ Breakfast		🍔 Lunch		✗ Dinner		🛏 Bedtime
	Time	Level	Time	Level	Time	Level	Time	Level
Pre								
Pos								

Notes:

Date:		Day:			Mood:		
	☕ Breakfast		🍔 Lunch		✗ Dinner		🛏 Bedtime
	Time	Level	Time	Level	Time	Level	Time	Level
Pre								
Pos								

Notes:

Date:		Day:			Mood:		
	☕ Breakfast		🍔 Lunch		✗ Dinner		🛏 Bedtime
	Time	Level	Time	Level	Time	Level	Time	Level
Pre								
Pos								

Notes:

Date:		Day:			Mood:		
	☕ Breakfast		🍔 Lunch		✗ Dinner		🛏 Bedtime
	Time	Level	Time	Level	Time	Level	Time	Level
Pre								
Pos								

Notes:

Date:			Day:			Mood:		
	🍵 Breakfast		🍔 Lunch		✗ Dinner		🛏 Bedtime	
	Time	Level	Time	Level	Time	Level	Time	Level
Pre								
Pos								
Notes:								

Date:			Day:			Mood:		
	🍵 Breakfast		🍔 Lunch		✗ Dinner		🛏 Bedtime	
	Time	Level	Time	Level	Time	Level	Time	Level
Pre								
Pos								
Notes:								

Date:			Day:			Mood:		
	🍵 Breakfast		🍔 Lunch		✗ Dinner		🛏 Bedtime	
	Time	Level	Time	Level	Time	Level	Time	Level
Pre								
Pos								
Notes:								

Date:			Day:			Mood:		
	🍵 Breakfast		🍔 Lunch		✗ Dinner		🛏 Bedtime	
	Time	Level	Time	Level	Time	Level	Time	Level
Pre								
Pos								
Notes:								

Date:			Day:			Mood:		
	🍵 Breakfast		🍔 Lunch		✗ Dinner		🛏 Bedtime	
	Time	Level	Time	Level	Time	Level	Time	Level
Pre								
Pos								
Notes:								

Date:			Day:			Mood:		
	🍵 Breakfast		🍔 Lunch		✗ Dinner		🛏 Bedtime	
	Time	Level	Time	Level	Time	Level	Time	Level
Pre								
Pos								
Notes:								

Date:				Day:			Mood:		
	☕ Breakfast		🍴 Lunch		✗ Dinner		🛏 Bedtime		
	Time	Level	Time	Level	Time	Level	Time	Level
Pre								
Pos								
Notes:								

Date:				Day:			Mood:		
	☕ Breakfast		🍴 Lunch		✗ Dinner		🛏 Bedtime		
	Time	Level	Time	Level	Time	Level	Time	Level
Pre								
Pos								
Notes:								

Date:				Day:			Mood:		
	☕ Breakfast		🍴 Lunch		✗ Dinner		🛏 Bedtime		
	Time	Level	Time	Level	Time	Level	Time	Level
Pre								
Pos								
Notes:								

Date:				Day:			Mood:		
	☕ Breakfast		🍴 Lunch		✗ Dinner		🛏 Bedtime		
	Time	Level	Time	Level	Time	Level	Time	Level
Pre								
Pos								
Notes:								

Date:				Day:			Mood:		
	☕ Breakfast		🍴 Lunch		✗ Dinner		🛏 Bedtime		
	Time	Level	Time	Level	Time	Level	Time	Level
Pre								
Pos								
Notes:								

Date:				Day:			Mood:		
	☕ Breakfast		🍴 Lunch		✗ Dinner		🛏 Bedtime		
	Time	Level	Time	Level	Time	Level	Time	Level
Pre								
Pos								
Notes:								

Date:			Day:			Mood:		
	☕ Breakfast		🍴 Lunch		✗ Dinner		🛏 Bedtime	
	Time	Level	Time	Level	Time	Level	Time	Level
Pre								
Pos								

Notes:

Date:			Day:			Mood:		
	☕ Breakfast		🍴 Lunch		✗ Dinner		🛏 Bedtime	
	Time	Level	Time	Level	Time	Level	Time	Level
Pre								
Pos								

Notes:

Date:			Day:			Mood:		
	☕ Breakfast		🍴 Lunch		✗ Dinner		🛏 Bedtime	
	Time	Level	Time	Level	Time	Level	Time	Level
Pre								
Pos								

Notes:

Date:			Day:			Mood:		
	☕ Breakfast		🍴 Lunch		✗ Dinner		🛏 Bedtime	
	Time	Level	Time	Level	Time	Level	Time	Level
Pre								
Pos								

Notes:

Date:			Day:			Mood:		
	☕ Breakfast		🍴 Lunch		✗ Dinner		🛏 Bedtime	
	Time	Level	Time	Level	Time	Level	Time	Level
Pre								
Pos								

Notes:

Date:			Day:			Mood:		
	☕ Breakfast		🍴 Lunch		✗ Dinner		🛏 Bedtime	
	Time	Level	Time	Level	Time	Level	Time	Level
Pre								
Pos								

Notes:

Date:			Day:			Mood:		
	☕ Breakfast		🍔 Lunch		✗ Dinner		🛏 Bedtime	
	Time	Level	Time	Level	Time	Level	Time	Level
Pre								
Pos								

Notes:

Date:			Day:			Mood:		
	☕ Breakfast		🍔 Lunch		✗ Dinner		🛏 Bedtime	
	Time	Level	Time	Level	Time	Level	Time	Level
Pre								
Pos								

Notes:

Date:			Day:			Mood:		
	☕ Breakfast		🍔 Lunch		✗ Dinner		🛏 Bedtime	
	Time	Level	Time	Level	Time	Level	Time	Level
Pre								
Pos								

Notes:

Date:			Day:			Mood:		
	☕ Breakfast		🍔 Lunch		✗ Dinner		🛏 Bedtime	
	Time	Level	Time	Level	Time	Level	Time	Level
Pre								
Pos								

Notes:

Date:			Day:			Mood:		
	☕ Breakfast		🍔 Lunch		✗ Dinner		🛏 Bedtime	
	Time	Level	Time	Level	Time	Level	Time	Level
Pre								
Pos								

Notes:

Date:			Day:			Mood:		
	☕ Breakfast		🍔 Lunch		✗ Dinner		🛏 Bedtime	
	Time	Level	Time	Level	Time	Level	Time	Level
Pre								
Pos								

Notes:

Date:			Day:			Mood:		
	☕ Breakfast		🍽 Lunch		✕ Dinner		🛏 Bedtime	
	Time	Level	Time	Level	Time	Level	Time	Level
Pre								
Pos								

Notes:

Date:			Day:			Mood:		
	☕ Breakfast		🍽 Lunch		✕ Dinner		🛏 Bedtime	
	Time	Level	Time	Level	Time	Level	Time	Level
Pre								
Pos								

Notes:

Date:			Day:			Mood:		
	☕ Breakfast		🍽 Lunch		✕ Dinner		🛏 Bedtime	
	Time	Level	Time	Level	Time	Level	Time	Level
Pre								
Pos								

Notes:

Date:			Day:			Mood:		
	☕ Breakfast		🍽 Lunch		✕ Dinner		🛏 Bedtime	
	Time	Level	Time	Level	Time	Level	Time	Level
Pre								
Pos								

Notes:

Date:			Day:			Mood:		
	☕ Breakfast		🍽 Lunch		✕ Dinner		🛏 Bedtime	
	Time	Level	Time	Level	Time	Level	Time	Level
Pre								
Pos								

Notes:

Date:			Day:			Mood:		
	☕ Breakfast		🍽 Lunch		✕ Dinner		🛏 Bedtime	
	Time	Level	Time	Level	Time	Level	Time	Level
Pre								
Pos								

Notes:

Date:		Day:			Mood:		
	☕ Breakfast		🍴 Lunch		✕ Dinner		🛏 Bedtime
	Time	Level	Time	Level	Time	Level	Time	Level
Pre								
Pos								

Notes:

Date:		Day:			Mood:		
	☕ Breakfast		🍴 Lunch		✕ Dinner		🛏 Bedtime
	Time	Level	Time	Level	Time	Level	Time	Level
Pre								
Pos								

Notes:

Date:		Day:			Mood:		
	☕ Breakfast		🍴 Lunch		✕ Dinner		🛏 Bedtime
	Time	Level	Time	Level	Time	Level	Time	Level
Pre								
Pos								

Notes:

Date:		Day:			Mood:		
	☕ Breakfast		🍴 Lunch		✕ Dinner		🛏 Bedtime
	Time	Level	Time	Level	Time	Level	Time	Level
Pre								
Pos								

Notes:

Date:		Day:			Mood:		
	☕ Breakfast		🍴 Lunch		✕ Dinner		🛏 Bedtime
	Time	Level	Time	Level	Time	Level	Time	Level
Pre								
Pos								

Notes:

Date:		Day:			Mood:		
	☕ Breakfast		🍴 Lunch		✕ Dinner		🛏 Bedtime
	Time	Level	Time	Level	Time	Level	Time	Level
Pre								
Pos								

Notes:

Date:			Day:			Mood:		
	☕ Breakfast		🍴 Lunch		✗ Dinner		🛏 Bedtime	
	Time	Level	Time	Level	Time	Level	Time	Level
Pre								
Pos								
Notes:								

Date:			Day:			Mood:		
	☕ Breakfast		🍴 Lunch		✗ Dinner		🛏 Bedtime	
	Time	Level	Time	Level	Time	Level	Time	Level
Pre								
Pos								
Notes:								

Date:			Day:			Mood:		
	☕ Breakfast		🍴 Lunch		✗ Dinner		🛏 Bedtime	
	Time	Level	Time	Level	Time	Level	Time	Level
Pre								
Pos								
Notes:								

Date:			Day:			Mood:		
	☕ Breakfast		🍴 Lunch		✗ Dinner		🛏 Bedtime	
	Time	Level	Time	Level	Time	Level	Time	Level
Pre								
Pos								
Notes:								

Date:			Day:			Mood:		
	☕ Breakfast		🍴 Lunch		✗ Dinner		🛏 Bedtime	
	Time	Level	Time	Level	Time	Level	Time	Level
Pre								
Pos								
Notes:								

Date:			Day:			Mood:		
	☕ Breakfast		🍴 Lunch		✗ Dinner		🛏 Bedtime	
	Time	Level	Time	Level	Time	Level	Time	Level
Pre								
Pos								
Notes:								

Date:			Day:			Mood:		
	☕ Breakfast		🍴 Lunch		✗ Dinner		🛏 Bedtime	
	Time	Level	Time	Level	Time	Level	Time	Level
Pre								
Pos								
Notes:								

Date:			Day:			Mood:		
	☕ Breakfast		🍴 Lunch		✗ Dinner		🛏 Bedtime	
	Time	Level	Time	Level	Time	Level	Time	Level
Pre								
Pos								
Notes:								

Date:			Day:			Mood:		
	☕ Breakfast		🍴 Lunch		✗ Dinner		🛏 Bedtime	
	Time	Level	Time	Level	Time	Level	Time	Level
Pre								
Pos								
Notes:								

Date:			Day:			Mood:		
	☕ Breakfast		🍴 Lunch		✗ Dinner		🛏 Bedtime	
	Time	Level	Time	Level	Time	Level	Time	Level
Pre								
Pos								
Notes:								

Date:			Day:			Mood:		
	☕ Breakfast		🍴 Lunch		✗ Dinner		🛏 Bedtime	
	Time	Level	Time	Level	Time	Level	Time	Level
Pre								
Pos								
Notes:								

Date:			Day:			Mood:		
	☕ Breakfast		🍴 Lunch		✗ Dinner		🛏 Bedtime	
	Time	Level	Time	Level	Time	Level	Time	Level
Pre								
Pos								
Notes:								

Date:			Day:			Mood:		
	☕ Breakfast		🍝 Lunch		✕ Dinner		🛏 Bedtime	
	Time	Level	Time	Level	Time	Level	Time	Level
Pre								
Pos								

Notes:

Date:			Day:			Mood:		
	☕ Breakfast		🍝 Lunch		✕ Dinner		🛏 Bedtime	
	Time	Level	Time	Level	Time	Level	Time	Level
Pre								
Pos								

Notes:

Date:			Day:			Mood:		
	☕ Breakfast		🍝 Lunch		✕ Dinner		🛏 Bedtime	
	Time	Level	Time	Level	Time	Level	Time	Level
Pre								
Pos								

Notes:

Date:			Day:			Mood:		
	☕ Breakfast		🍝 Lunch		✕ Dinner		🛏 Bedtime	
	Time	Level	Time	Level	Time	Level	Time	Level
Pre								
Pos								

Notes:

Date:			Day:			Mood:		
	☕ Breakfast		🍝 Lunch		✕ Dinner		🛏 Bedtime	
	Time	Level	Time	Level	Time	Level	Time	Level
Pre								
Pos								

Notes:

Date:			Day:			Mood:		
	☕ Breakfast		🍝 Lunch		✕ Dinner		🛏 Bedtime	
	Time	Level	Time	Level	Time	Level	Time	Level
Pre								
Pos								

Notes:

Date:			Day:			Mood:		
	☕ Breakfast		🍴 Lunch		✗ Dinner		🛏 Bedtime	
	Time	Level	Time	Level	Time	Level	Time	Level
Pre								
Pos								

Notes:

Date:			Day:			Mood:		
	☕ Breakfast		🍴 Lunch		✗ Dinner		🛏 Bedtime	
	Time	Level	Time	Level	Time	Level	Time	Level
Pre								
Pos								

Notes:

Date:			Day:			Mood:		
	☕ Breakfast		🍴 Lunch		✗ Dinner		🛏 Bedtime	
	Time	Level	Time	Level	Time	Level	Time	Level
Pre								
Pos								

Notes:

Date:			Day:			Mood:		
	☕ Breakfast		🍴 Lunch		✗ Dinner		🛏 Bedtime	
	Time	Level	Time	Level	Time	Level	Time	Level
Pre								
Pos								

Notes:

Date:			Day:			Mood:		
	☕ Breakfast		🍴 Lunch		✗ Dinner		🛏 Bedtime	
	Time	Level	Time	Level	Time	Level	Time	Level
Pre								
Pos								

Notes:

Date:			Day:			Mood:		
	☕ Breakfast		🍴 Lunch		✗ Dinner		🛏 Bedtime	
	Time	Level	Time	Level	Time	Level	Time	Level
Pre								
Pos								

Notes:

Date:			Day:			Mood:		
	☕ Breakfast		🍴 Lunch		✕ Dinner		🛏 Bedtime	
	Time	Level	Time	Level	Time	Level	Time	Level
Pre								
Pos								

Notes:

Date:			Day:			Mood:		
	☕ Breakfast		🍴 Lunch		✕ Dinner		🛏 Bedtime	
	Time	Level	Time	Level	Time	Level	Time	Level
Pre								
Pos								

Notes:

Date:			Day:			Mood:		
	☕ Breakfast		🍴 Lunch		✕ Dinner		🛏 Bedtime	
	Time	Level	Time	Level	Time	Level	Time	Level
Pre								
Pos								

Notes:

Date:			Day:			Mood:		
	☕ Breakfast		🍴 Lunch		✕ Dinner		🛏 Bedtime	
	Time	Level	Time	Level	Time	Level	Time	Level
Pre								
Pos								

Notes:

Date:			Day:			Mood:		
	☕ Breakfast		🍴 Lunch		✕ Dinner		🛏 Bedtime	
	Time	Level	Time	Level	Time	Level	Time	Level
Pre								
Pos								

Notes:

Date:			Day:			Mood:		
	☕ Breakfast		🍴 Lunch		✕ Dinner		🛏 Bedtime	
	Time	Level	Time	Level	Time	Level	Time	Level
Pre								
Pos								

Notes:

Date:			Day:			Mood:		
	☕ Breakfast		🍴 Lunch		✕ Dinner		🛏 Bedtime	
	Time	Level	Time	Level	Time	Level	Time	Level
Pre								
Pos								
Notes:								

Date:			Day:			Mood:		
	☕ Breakfast		🍴 Lunch		✕ Dinner		🛏 Bedtime	
	Time	Level	Time	Level	Time	Level	Time	Level
Pre								
Pos								
Notes:								

Date:			Day:			Mood:		
	☕ Breakfast		🍴 Lunch		✕ Dinner		🛏 Bedtime	
	Time	Level	Time	Level	Time	Level	Time	Level
Pre								
Pos								
Notes:								

Date:			Day:			Mood:		
	☕ Breakfast		🍴 Lunch		✕ Dinner		🛏 Bedtime	
	Time	Level	Time	Level	Time	Level	Time	Level
Pre								
Pos								
Notes:								

Date:			Day:			Mood:		
	☕ Breakfast		🍴 Lunch		✕ Dinner		🛏 Bedtime	
	Time	Level	Time	Level	Time	Level	Time	Level
Pre								
Pos								
Notes:								

Date:			Day:			Mood:		
	☕ Breakfast		🍴 Lunch		✕ Dinner		🛏 Bedtime	
	Time	Level	Time	Level	Time	Level	Time	Level
Pre								
Pos								
Notes:								

Date:			Day:			Mood:		
	☕ Breakfast		🍴 Lunch		✗ Dinner		🛏 Bedtime	
	Time	Level	Time	Level	Time	Level	Time	Level
Pre								
Pos								
Notes:								

Date:			Day:			Mood:		
	☕ Breakfast		🍴 Lunch		✗ Dinner		🛏 Bedtime	
	Time	Level	Time	Level	Time	Level	Time	Level
Pre								
Pos								
Notes:								

Date:			Day:			Mood:		
	☕ Breakfast		🍴 Lunch		✗ Dinner		🛏 Bedtime	
	Time	Level	Time	Level	Time	Level	Time	Level
Pre								
Pos								
Notes:								

Date:			Day:			Mood:		
	☕ Breakfast		🍴 Lunch		✗ Dinner		🛏 Bedtime	
	Time	Level	Time	Level	Time	Level	Time	Level
Pre								
Pos								
Notes:								

Date:			Day:			Mood:		
	☕ Breakfast		🍴 Lunch		✗ Dinner		🛏 Bedtime	
	Time	Level	Time	Level	Time	Level	Time	Level
Pre								
Pos								
Notes:								

Date:			Day:			Mood:		
	☕ Breakfast		🍴 Lunch		✗ Dinner		🛏 Bedtime	
	Time	Level	Time	Level	Time	Level	Time	Level
Pre								
Pos								
Notes:								

Date:		Day:		Mood:	

	Breakfast		Lunch		Dinner		Bedtime	
	Time	Level	Time	Level	Time	Level	Time	Level
Pre								
Pos								

Notes:

Date:		Day:		Mood:	

	Breakfast		Lunch		Dinner		Bedtime	
	Time	Level	Time	Level	Time	Level	Time	Level
Pre								
Pos								

Notes:

Date:		Day:		Mood:	

	Breakfast		Lunch		Dinner		Bedtime	
	Time	Level	Time	Level	Time	Level	Time	Level
Pre								
Pos								

Notes:

Date:		Day:		Mood:	

	Breakfast		Lunch		Dinner		Bedtime	
	Time	Level	Time	Level	Time	Level	Time	Level
Pre								
Pos								

Notes:

Date:		Day:		Mood:	

	Breakfast		Lunch		Dinner		Bedtime	
	Time	Level	Time	Level	Time	Level	Time	Level
Pre								
Pos								

Notes:

Date:		Day:		Mood:	

	Breakfast		Lunch		Dinner		Bedtime	
	Time	Level	Time	Level	Time	Level	Time	Level
Pre								
Pos								

Notes:

Date:			Day:			Mood:		
	☕ Breakfast		🍲 Lunch		✗ Dinner		🛏 Bedtime	
	Time	Level	Time	Level	Time	Level	Time	Level
Pre								
Pos								
Notes:								

Date:			Day:			Mood:		
	☕ Breakfast		🍲 Lunch		✗ Dinner		🛏 Bedtime	
	Time	Level	Time	Level	Time	Level	Time	Level
Pre								
Pos								
Notes:								

Date:			Day:			Mood:		
	☕ Breakfast		🍲 Lunch		✗ Dinner		🛏 Bedtime	
	Time	Level	Time	Level	Time	Level	Time	Level
Pre								
Pos								
Notes:								

Date:			Day:			Mood:		
	☕ Breakfast		🍲 Lunch		✗ Dinner		🛏 Bedtime	
	Time	Level	Time	Level	Time	Level	Time	Level
Pre								
Pos								
Notes:								

Date:			Day:			Mood:		
	☕ Breakfast		🍲 Lunch		✗ Dinner		🛏 Bedtime	
	Time	Level	Time	Level	Time	Level	Time	Level
Pre								
Pos								
Notes:								

Date:			Day:			Mood:		
	☕ Breakfast		🍲 Lunch		✗ Dinner		🛏 Bedtime	
	Time	Level	Time	Level	Time	Level	Time	Level
Pre								
Pos								
Notes:								

Date:			Day:			Mood:			
	🍵 Breakfast		🍚 Lunch		✗ Dinner		🛏 Bedtime		
	Time	Level	Time	Level	Time	Level	Time	Level
Pre								
Pos								
Notes:									

Date:			Day:			Mood:			
	🍵 Breakfast		🍚 Lunch		✗ Dinner		🛏 Bedtime		
	Time	Level	Time	Level	Time	Level	Time	Level
Pre								
Pos								
Notes:									

Date:			Day:			Mood:			
	🍵 Breakfast		🍚 Lunch		✗ Dinner		🛏 Bedtime		
	Time	Level	Time	Level	Time	Level	Time	Level
Pre								
Pos								
Notes:									

Date:			Day:			Mood:			
	🍵 Breakfast		🍚 Lunch		✗ Dinner		🛏 Bedtime		
	Time	Level	Time	Level	Time	Level	Time	Level
Pre								
Pos								
Notes:									

Date:			Day:			Mood:			
	🍵 Breakfast		🍚 Lunch		✗ Dinner		🛏 Bedtime		
	Time	Level	Time	Level	Time	Level	Time	Level
Pre								
Pos								
Notes:									

Date:			Day:			Mood:			
	🍵 Breakfast		🍚 Lunch		✗ Dinner		🛏 Bedtime		
	Time	Level	Time	Level	Time	Level	Time	Level
Pre								
Pos								
Notes:									

Date:		Day:			Mood:		
	☕ Breakfast		🍲 Lunch		✗ Dinner		🛏 Bedtime
	Time	Level	Time	Level	Time	Level	Time	Level
Pre								
Pos								

Notes:

Date:		Day:			Mood:		
	☕ Breakfast		🍲 Lunch		✗ Dinner		🛏 Bedtime
	Time	Level	Time	Level	Time	Level	Time	Level
Pre								
Pos								

Notes:

Date:		Day:			Mood:		
	☕ Breakfast		🍲 Lunch		✗ Dinner		🛏 Bedtime
	Time	Level	Time	Level	Time	Level	Time	Level
Pre								
Pos								

Notes:

Date:		Day:			Mood:		
	☕ Breakfast		🍲 Lunch		✗ Dinner		🛏 Bedtime
	Time	Level	Time	Level	Time	Level	Time	Level
Pre								
Pos								

Notes:

Date:		Day:			Mood:		
	☕ Breakfast		🍲 Lunch		✗ Dinner		🛏 Bedtime
	Time	Level	Time	Level	Time	Level	Time	Level
Pre								
Pos								

Notes:

Date:		Day:			Mood:		
	☕ Breakfast		🍲 Lunch		✗ Dinner		🛏 Bedtime
	Time	Level	Time	Level	Time	Level	Time	Level
Pre								
Pos								

Notes:

Date:			Day:				Mood:		
	☕ Breakfast		🍴 Lunch		✗ Dinner		🛏 Bedtime		
	Time	Level	Time	Level	Time	Level	Time	Level
Pre								
Pos								
Notes:									

Date:			Day:				Mood:		
	☕ Breakfast		🍴 Lunch		✗ Dinner		🛏 Bedtime		
	Time	Level	Time	Level	Time	Level	Time	Level
Pre								
Pos								
Notes:									

Date:			Day:				Mood:		
	☕ Breakfast		🍴 Lunch		✗ Dinner		🛏 Bedtime		
	Time	Level	Time	Level	Time	Level	Time	Level
Pre								
Pos								
Notes:									

Date:			Day:				Mood:		
	☕ Breakfast		🍴 Lunch		✗ Dinner		🛏 Bedtime		
	Time	Level	Time	Level	Time	Level	Time	Level
Pre								
Pos								
Notes:									

Date:			Day:				Mood:		
	☕ Breakfast		🍴 Lunch		✗ Dinner		🛏 Bedtime		
	Time	Level	Time	Level	Time	Level	Time	Level
Pre								
Pos								
Notes:									

Date:			Day:				Mood:		
	☕ Breakfast		🍴 Lunch		✗ Dinner		🛏 Bedtime		
	Time	Level	Time	Level	Time	Level	Time	Level
Pre								
Pos								
Notes:									

Date:			Day:			Mood:		
	☕ Breakfast		🍲 Lunch		✗ Dinner		🛏 Bedtime	
	Time	Level	Time	Level	Time	Level	Time	Level
Pre								
Pos								

Notes:

Date:			Day:			Mood:		
	☕ Breakfast		🍲 Lunch		✗ Dinner		🛏 Bedtime	
	Time	Level	Time	Level	Time	Level	Time	Level
Pre								
Pos								

Notes:

Date:			Day:			Mood:		
	☕ Breakfast		🍲 Lunch		✗ Dinner		🛏 Bedtime	
	Time	Level	Time	Level	Time	Level	Time	Level
Pre								
Pos								

Notes:

Date:			Day:			Mood:		
	☕ Breakfast		🍲 Lunch		✗ Dinner		🛏 Bedtime	
	Time	Level	Time	Level	Time	Level	Time	Level
Pre								
Pos								

Notes:

Date:			Day:			Mood:		
	☕ Breakfast		🍲 Lunch		✗ Dinner		🛏 Bedtime	
	Time	Level	Time	Level	Time	Level	Time	Level
Pre								
Pos								

Notes:

Date:			Day:			Mood:		
	☕ Breakfast		🍲 Lunch		✗ Dinner		🛏 Bedtime	
	Time	Level	Time	Level	Time	Level	Time	Level
Pre								
Pos								

Notes:

Date:		Day:			Mood:			
	☕ **Breakfast**		🍲 **Lunch**		✗ **Dinner**		🛏 **Bedtime**	
	Time	Level	Time	Level	Time	Level	Time	Level
Pre								
Pos								
Notes:								

Date:		Day:			Mood:			
	☕ **Breakfast**		🍲 **Lunch**		✗ **Dinner**		🛏 **Bedtime**	
	Time	Level	Time	Level	Time	Level	Time	Level
Pre								
Pos								
Notes:								

Date:		Day:			Mood:			
	☕ **Breakfast**		🍲 **Lunch**		✗ **Dinner**		🛏 **Bedtime**	
	Time	Level	Time	Level	Time	Level	Time	Level
Pre								
Pos								
Notes:								

Date:		Day:			Mood:			
	☕ **Breakfast**		🍲 **Lunch**		✗ **Dinner**		🛏 **Bedtime**	
	Time	Level	Time	Level	Time	Level	Time	Level
Pre								
Pos								
Notes:								

Date:		Day:			Mood:			
	☕ **Breakfast**		🍲 **Lunch**		✗ **Dinner**		🛏 **Bedtime**	
	Time	Level	Time	Level	Time	Level	Time	Level
Pre								
Pos								
Notes:								

Date:		Day:			Mood:			
	☕ **Breakfast**		🍲 **Lunch**		✗ **Dinner**		🛏 **Bedtime**	
	Time	Level	Time	Level	Time	Level	Time	Level
Pre								
Pos								
Notes:								

Date:			Day:			Mood:			
	🍵 Breakfast		🍝 Lunch		✕ Dinner		🛏 Bedtime		
	Time	Level	Time	Level	Time	Level	Time	Level
re								
os								

Notes:

Date:			Day:			Mood:			
	🍵 Breakfast		🍝 Lunch		✕ Dinner		🛏 Bedtime		
	Time	Level	Time	Level	Time	Level	Time	Level
re								
os								

Notes:

Date:			Day:			Mood:			
	🍵 Breakfast		🍝 Lunch		✕ Dinner		🛏 Bedtime		
	Time	Level	Time	Level	Time	Level	Time	Level
re								
os								

Notes:

Date:			Day:			Mood:			
	🍵 Breakfast		🍝 Lunch		✕ Dinner		🛏 Bedtime		
	Time	Level	Time	Level	Time	Level	Time	Level
re								
os								

Notes:

Date:			Day:			Mood:			
	🍵 Breakfast		🍝 Lunch		✕ Dinner		🛏 Bedtime		
	Time	Level	Time	Level	Time	Level	Time	Level
re								
os								

Notes:

Date:			Day:			Mood:			
	🍵 Breakfast		🍝 Lunch		✕ Dinner		🛏 Bedtime		
	Time	Level	Time	Level	Time	Level	Time	Level
re								
os								

Notes:

Date:			Day:			Mood:			
	☕ Breakfast		🍴 Lunch		✗ Dinner		🛏 Bedtime		
	Time	Level	Time	Level	Time	Level	Time	Level
Pre								
Pos								
Notes:								

Date:			Day:			Mood:			
	☕ Breakfast		🍴 Lunch		✗ Dinner		🛏 Bedtime		
	Time	Level	Time	Level	Time	Level	Time	Level
Pre								
Pos								
Notes:								

Date:			Day:			Mood:			
	☕ Breakfast		🍴 Lunch		✗ Dinner		🛏 Bedtime		
	Time	Level	Time	Level	Time	Level	Time	Level
Pre								
Pos								
Notes:								

Date:			Day:			Mood:			
	☕ Breakfast		🍴 Lunch		✗ Dinner		🛏 Bedtime		
	Time	Level	Time	Level	Time	Level	Time	Level
Pre								
Pos								
Notes:								

Date:			Day:			Mood:			
	☕ Breakfast		🍴 Lunch		✗ Dinner		🛏 Bedtime		
	Time	Level	Time	Level	Time	Level	Time	Level
Pre								
Pos								
Notes:								

Date:			Day:			Mood:			
	☕ Breakfast		🍴 Lunch		✗ Dinner		🛏 Bedtime		
	Time	Level	Time	Level	Time	Level	Time	Level
Pre								
Pos								
Notes:								

Date:			Day:			Mood:		
	☕ Breakfast		🍲 Lunch		✕ Dinner		🛏 Bedtime	
	Time	Level	Time	Level	Time	Level	Time	Level
Pre								
Pos								

Notes:

Date:			Day:			Mood:		
	☕ Breakfast		🍲 Lunch		✕ Dinner		🛏 Bedtime	
	Time	Level	Time	Level	Time	Level	Time	Level
Pre								
Pos								

Notes:

Date:			Day:			Mood:		
	☕ Breakfast		🍲 Lunch		✕ Dinner		🛏 Bedtime	
	Time	Level	Time	Level	Time	Level	Time	Level
Pre								
Pos								

Notes:

Date:			Day:			Mood:		
	☕ Breakfast		🍲 Lunch		✕ Dinner		🛏 Bedtime	
	Time	Level	Time	Level	Time	Level	Time	Level
Pre								
Pos								

Notes:

Date:			Day:			Mood:		
	☕ Breakfast		🍲 Lunch		✕ Dinner		🛏 Bedtime	
	Time	Level	Time	Level	Time	Level	Time	Level
Pre								
Pos								

Notes:

Date:			Day:			Mood:		
	☕ Breakfast		🍲 Lunch		✕ Dinner		🛏 Bedtime	
	Time	Level	Time	Level	Time	Level	Time	Level
Pre								
Pos								

Notes:

Date:			Day:			Mood:		
	☕ Breakfast		🍵 Lunch		✗ Dinner		🛏 Bedtime	
	Time	Level	Time	Level	Time	Level	Time	Level
Pre								
Pos								
Notes:								

Date:			Day:			Mood:		
	☕ Breakfast		🍵 Lunch		✗ Dinner		🛏 Bedtime	
	Time	Level	Time	Level	Time	Level	Time	Level
Pre								
Pos								
Notes:								

Date:			Day:			Mood:		
	☕ Breakfast		🍵 Lunch		✗ Dinner		🛏 Bedtime	
	Time	Level	Time	Level	Time	Level	Time	Level
Pre								
Pos								
Notes:								

Date:			Day:			Mood:		
	☕ Breakfast		🍵 Lunch		✗ Dinner		🛏 Bedtime	
	Time	Level	Time	Level	Time	Level	Time	Level
Pre								
Pos								
Notes:								

Date:			Day:			Mood:		
	☕ Breakfast		🍵 Lunch		✗ Dinner		🛏 Bedtime	
	Time	Level	Time	Level	Time	Level	Time	Level
Pre								
Pos								
Notes:								

Date:			Day:			Mood:		
	☕ Breakfast		🍵 Lunch		✗ Dinner		🛏 Bedtime	
	Time	Level	Time	Level	Time	Level	Time	Level
Pre								
Pos								
Notes:								

Date:			Day:			Mood:		
	🍵 Breakfast		🍝 Lunch		✗ Dinner		🛏 Bedtime	
	Time	Level	Time	Level	Time	Level	Time	Level
re								
os								

Notes:

Date:			Day:			Mood:		
	🍵 Breakfast		🍝 Lunch		✗ Dinner		🛏 Bedtime	
	Time	Level	Time	Level	Time	Level	Time	Level
re								
os								

Notes:

Date:			Day:			Mood:		
	🍵 Breakfast		🍝 Lunch		✗ Dinner		🛏 Bedtime	
	Time	Level	Time	Level	Time	Level	Time	Level
re								
os								

Notes:

Date:			Day:			Mood:		
	🍵 Breakfast		🍝 Lunch		✗ Dinner		🛏 Bedtime	
	Time	Level	Time	Level	Time	Level	Time	Level
re								
os								

Notes:

Date:			Day:			Mood:		
	🍵 Breakfast		🍝 Lunch		✗ Dinner		🛏 Bedtime	
	Time	Level	Time	Level	Time	Level	Time	Level
re								
os								

Notes:

Date:			Day:			Mood:		
	🍵 Breakfast		🍝 Lunch		✗ Dinner		🛏 Bedtime	
	Time	Level	Time	Level	Time	Level	Time	Level
re								
os								

Notes:

Date:			Day:			Mood:		
	☕ Breakfast		🍴 Lunch		✗ Dinner		🛏 Bedtime	
	Time	Level	Time	Level	Time	Level	Time	Level
Pre								
Pos								

Notes:

Date:			Day:			Mood:		
	☕ Breakfast		🍴 Lunch		✗ Dinner		🛏 Bedtime	
	Time	Level	Time	Level	Time	Level	Time	Level
Pre								
Pos								

Notes:

Date:			Day:			Mood:		
	☕ Breakfast		🍴 Lunch		✗ Dinner		🛏 Bedtime	
	Time	Level	Time	Level	Time	Level	Time	Level
Pre								
Pos								

Notes:

Date:			Day:			Mood:		
	☕ Breakfast		🍴 Lunch		✗ Dinner		🛏 Bedtime	
	Time	Level	Time	Level	Time	Level	Time	Level
Pre								
Pos								

Notes:

Date:			Day:			Mood:		
	☕ Breakfast		🍴 Lunch		✗ Dinner		🛏 Bedtime	
	Time	Level	Time	Level	Time	Level	Time	Level
Pre								
Pos								

Notes:

Date:			Day:			Mood:		
	☕ Breakfast		🍴 Lunch		✗ Dinner		🛏 Bedtime	
	Time	Level	Time	Level	Time	Level	Time	Level
Pre								
Pos								

Notes:

Date:			Day:			Mood:		
	☕ Breakfast		🍴 Lunch		✕ Dinner		🛏 Bedtime	
	Time	Level	Time	Level	Time	Level	Time	Level
re								
os								

Notes:

Date:			Day:			Mood:		
	☕ Breakfast		🍴 Lunch		✕ Dinner		🛏 Bedtime	
	Time	Level	Time	Level	Time	Level	Time	Level
re								
os								

Notes:

Date:			Day:			Mood:		
	☕ Breakfast		🍴 Lunch		✕ Dinner		🛏 Bedtime	
	Time	Level	Time	Level	Time	Level	Time	Level
re								
os								

Notes:

Date:			Day:			Mood:		
	☕ Breakfast		🍴 Lunch		✕ Dinner		🛏 Bedtime	
	Time	Level	Time	Level	Time	Level	Time	Level
re								
os								

Notes:

Date:			Day:			Mood:		
	☕ Breakfast		🍴 Lunch		✕ Dinner		🛏 Bedtime	
	Time	Level	Time	Level	Time	Level	Time	Level
re								
os								

Notes:

Date:			Day:			Mood:		
	☕ Breakfast		🍴 Lunch		✕ Dinner		🛏 Bedtime	
	Time	Level	Time	Level	Time	Level	Time	Level
re								
os								

Notes:

Date:			Day:			Mood:		
	☕ Breakfast		🍴 Lunch		✕ Dinner		🛏 Bedtime	
	Time	Level	Time	Level	Time	Level	Time	Level
Pre								
Pos								

Notes:

Date:			Day:			Mood:		
	☕ Breakfast		🍴 Lunch		✕ Dinner		🛏 Bedtime	
	Time	Level	Time	Level	Time	Level	Time	Level
Pre								
Pos								

Notes:

Date:			Day:			Mood:		
	☕ Breakfast		🍴 Lunch		✕ Dinner		🛏 Bedtime	
	Time	Level	Time	Level	Time	Level	Time	Level
Pre								
Pos								

Notes:

Date:			Day:			Mood:		
	☕ Breakfast		🍴 Lunch		✕ Dinner		🛏 Bedtime	
	Time	Level	Time	Level	Time	Level	Time	Level
Pre								
Pos								

Notes:

Date:			Day:			Mood:		
	☕ Breakfast		🍴 Lunch		✕ Dinner		🛏 Bedtime	
	Time	Level	Time	Level	Time	Level	Time	Level
Pre								
Pos								

Notes:

Date:			Day:			Mood:		
	☕ Breakfast		🍴 Lunch		✕ Dinner		🛏 Bedtime	
	Time	Level	Time	Level	Time	Level	Time	Level
Pre								
Pos								

Notes:

Date:		Day:			Mood:		
	🍵 Breakfast		🍴 Lunch		✗ Dinner		🛏 Bedtime
	Time	Level	Time	Level	Time	Level	Time	Level
re								
os								

Notes:

Date:		Day:			Mood:		
	🍵 Breakfast		🍴 Lunch		✗ Dinner		🛏 Bedtime
	Time	Level	Time	Level	Time	Level	Time	Level
re								
os								

Notes:

Date:		Day:			Mood:		
	🍵 Breakfast		🍴 Lunch		✗ Dinner		🛏 Bedtime
	Time	Level	Time	Level	Time	Level	Time	Level
re								
os								

Notes:

Date:		Day:			Mood:		
	🍵 Breakfast		🍴 Lunch		✗ Dinner		🛏 Bedtime
	Time	Level	Time	Level	Time	Level	Time	Level
re								
os								

Notes:

Date:		Day:			Mood:		
	🍵 Breakfast		🍴 Lunch		✗ Dinner		🛏 Bedtime
	Time	Level	Time	Level	Time	Level	Time	Level
re								
os								

Notes:

Date:		Day:			Mood:		
	🍵 Breakfast		🍴 Lunch		✗ Dinner		🛏 Bedtime
	Time	Level	Time	Level	Time	Level	Time	Level
re								
os								

Notes:

Date:			Day:			Mood:			
	☕ Breakfast		🍴 Lunch		✗ Dinner		🛏 Bedtime		
	Time	Level	Time	Level	Time	Level	Time	Level
Pre								
Pos								
Notes:								

Date:			Day:			Mood:			
	☕ Breakfast		🍴 Lunch		✗ Dinner		🛏 Bedtime		
	Time	Level	Time	Level	Time	Level	Time	Level
Pre								
Pos								
Notes:								

Date:			Day:			Mood:			
	☕ Breakfast		🍴 Lunch		✗ Dinner		🛏 Bedtime		
	Time	Level	Time	Level	Time	Level	Time	Level
Pre								
Pos								
Notes:								

Date:			Day:			Mood:			
	☕ Breakfast		🍴 Lunch		✗ Dinner		🛏 Bedtime		
	Time	Level	Time	Level	Time	Level	Time	Level
Pre								
Pos								
Notes:								

Date:			Day:			Mood:			
	☕ Breakfast		🍴 Lunch		✗ Dinner		🛏 Bedtime		
	Time	Level	Time	Level	Time	Level	Time	Level
Pre								
Pos								
Notes:								

Date:			Day:			Mood:			
	☕ Breakfast		🍴 Lunch		✗ Dinner		🛏 Bedtime		
	Time	Level	Time	Level	Time	Level	Time	Level
Pre								
Pos								
Notes:								

Date:			Day:			Mood:		
	🍵 Breakfast		🍴 Lunch		✗ Dinner		🛏 Bedtime	
	Time	Level	Time	Level	Time	Level	Time	Level
re								
os								
Notes:								

Date:			Day:			Mood:		
	🍵 Breakfast		🍴 Lunch		✗ Dinner		🛏 Bedtime	
	Time	Level	Time	Level	Time	Level	Time	Level
re								
os								
Notes:								

Date:			Day:			Mood:		
	🍵 Breakfast		🍴 Lunch		✗ Dinner		🛏 Bedtime	
	Time	Level	Time	Level	Time	Level	Time	Level
re								
os								
Notes:								

Date:			Day:			Mood:		
	🍵 Breakfast		🍴 Lunch		✗ Dinner		🛏 Bedtime	
	Time	Level	Time	Level	Time	Level	Time	Level
re								
os								
Notes:								

Date:			Day:			Mood:		
	🍵 Breakfast		🍴 Lunch		✗ Dinner		🛏 Bedtime	
	Time	Level	Time	Level	Time	Level	Time	Level
re								
os								
Notes:								

Date:			Day:			Mood:		
	🍵 Breakfast		🍴 Lunch		✗ Dinner		🛏 Bedtime	
	Time	Level	Time	Level	Time	Level	Time	Level
re								
os								
Notes:								

Date:			Day:			Mood:		
☕ Breakfast		🍴 Lunch		✗ Dinner		🛏 Bedtime		
Time	Level	Time	Level	Time	Level	Time	Level
Pre								
Pos								

Notes:

Date:			Day:			Mood:		
☕ Breakfast		🍴 Lunch		✗ Dinner		🛏 Bedtime		
Time	Level	Time	Level	Time	Level	Time	Level
Pre								
Pos								

Notes:

Date:			Day:			Mood:		
☕ Breakfast		🍴 Lunch		✗ Dinner		🛏 Bedtime		
Time	Level	Time	Level	Time	Level	Time	Level
Pre								
Pos								

Notes:

Date:			Day:			Mood:		
☕ Breakfast		🍴 Lunch		✗ Dinner		🛏 Bedtime		
Time	Level	Time	Level	Time	Level	Time	Level
Pre								
Pos								

Notes:

Date:			Day:			Mood:		
☕ Breakfast		🍴 Lunch		✗ Dinner		🛏 Bedtime		
Time	Level	Time	Level	Time	Level	Time	Level
Pre								
Pos								

Notes:

Date:			Day:			Mood:		
☕ Breakfast		🍴 Lunch		✗ Dinner		🛏 Bedtime		
Time	Level	Time	Level	Time	Level	Time	Level
Pre								
Pos								

Notes:

Date:			Day:			Mood:		
	☕ Breakfast		🍴 Lunch		✗ Dinner		🛏 Bedtime	
	Time	Level	Time	Level	Time	Level	Time	Level
're								
'os								
Notes:								

Date:			Day:			Mood:		
	☕ Breakfast		🍴 Lunch		✗ Dinner		🛏 Bedtime	
	Time	Level	Time	Level	Time	Level	Time	Level
're								
'os								
Notes:								

Date:			Day:			Mood:		
	☕ Breakfast		🍴 Lunch		✗ Dinner		🛏 Bedtime	
	Time	Level	Time	Level	Time	Level	Time	Level
're								
'os								
Notes:								

Date:			Day:			Mood:		
	☕ Breakfast		🍴 Lunch		✗ Dinner		🛏 Bedtime	
	Time	Level	Time	Level	Time	Level	Time	Level
're								
'os								
Notes:								

Date:			Day:			Mood:		
	☕ Breakfast		🍴 Lunch		✗ Dinner		🛏 Bedtime	
	Time	Level	Time	Level	Time	Level	Time	Level
're								
'os								
Notes:								

Date:			Day:			Mood:		
	☕ Breakfast		🍴 Lunch		✗ Dinner		🛏 Bedtime	
	Time	Level	Time	Level	Time	Level	Time	Level
're								
'os								
Notes:								

Date:		Day:			Mood:		
	☕ Breakfast		🍴 Lunch		✗ Dinner		🛏 Bedtime
	Time	Level	Time	Level	Time	Level	Time	Level
Pre								
Pos								

Notes:

Date:		Day:			Mood:		
	☕ Breakfast		🍴 Lunch		✗ Dinner		🛏 Bedtime
	Time	Level	Time	Level	Time	Level	Time	Level
Pre								
Pos								

Notes:

Date:		Day:			Mood:		
	☕ Breakfast		🍴 Lunch		✗ Dinner		🛏 Bedtime
	Time	Level	Time	Level	Time	Level	Time	Level
Pre								
Pos								

Notes:

Date:		Day:			Mood:		
	☕ Breakfast		🍴 Lunch		✗ Dinner		🛏 Bedtime
	Time	Level	Time	Level	Time	Level	Time	Level
Pre								
Pos								

Notes:

Date:		Day:			Mood:		
	☕ Breakfast		🍴 Lunch		✗ Dinner		🛏 Bedtime
	Time	Level	Time	Level	Time	Level	Time	Level
Pre								
Pos								

Notes:

Date:		Day:			Mood:		
	☕ Breakfast		🍴 Lunch		✗ Dinner		🛏 Bedtime
	Time	Level	Time	Level	Time	Level	Time	Level
Pre								
Pos								

Notes:

Date:		Day:			Mood:			
	🍵 Breakfast		🍝 Lunch		✗ Dinner		🛏 Bedtime	
	Time	Level	Time	Level	Time	Level	Time	Level
re								
os								

Notes:

Date:		Day:			Mood:			
	🍵 Breakfast		🍝 Lunch		✗ Dinner		🛏 Bedtime	
	Time	Level	Time	Level	Time	Level	Time	Level
re								
os								

Notes:

Date:		Day:			Mood:			
	🍵 Breakfast		🍝 Lunch		✗ Dinner		🛏 Bedtime	
	Time	Level	Time	Level	Time	Level	Time	Level
re								
os								

Notes:

Date:		Day:			Mood:			
	🍵 Breakfast		🍝 Lunch		✗ Dinner		🛏 Bedtime	
	Time	Level	Time	Level	Time	Level	Time	Level
re								
os								

Notes:

Date:		Day:			Mood:			
	🍵 Breakfast		🍝 Lunch		✗ Dinner		🛏 Bedtime	
	Time	Level	Time	Level	Time	Level	Time	Level
re								
os								

Notes:

Date:		Day:			Mood:			
	🍵 Breakfast		🍝 Lunch		✗ Dinner		🛏 Bedtime	
	Time	Level	Time	Level	Time	Level	Time	Level
re								
os								

Notes:

Date:			Day:			Mood:		
	☕ Breakfast		🍲 Lunch		✕ Dinner		🛏 Bedtime	
	Time	Level	Time	Level	Time	Level	Time	Level
Pre								
Pos								
Notes:								

Date:			Day:			Mood:		
	☕ Breakfast		🍲 Lunch		✕ Dinner		🛏 Bedtime	
	Time	Level	Time	Level	Time	Level	Time	Level
Pre								
Pos								
Notes:								

Date:			Day:			Mood:		
	☕ Breakfast		🍲 Lunch		✕ Dinner		🛏 Bedtime	
	Time	Level	Time	Level	Time	Level	Time	Level
Pre								
Pos								
Notes:								

Date:			Day:			Mood:		
	☕ Breakfast		🍲 Lunch		✕ Dinner		🛏 Bedtime	
	Time	Level	Time	Level	Time	Level	Time	Level
Pre								
Pos								
Notes:								

Date:			Day:			Mood:		
	☕ Breakfast		🍲 Lunch		✕ Dinner		🛏 Bedtime	
	Time	Level	Time	Level	Time	Level	Time	Level
Pre								
Pos								
Notes:								

Date:			Day:			Mood:		
	☕ Breakfast		🍲 Lunch		✕ Dinner		🛏 Bedtime	
	Time	Level	Time	Level	Time	Level	Time	Level
Pre								
Pos								
Notes:								

Date:			Day:			Mood:		
	🍵 Breakfast		🍝 Lunch		✗ Dinner		🛏 Bedtime	
	Time	Level	Time	Level	Time	Level	Time	Level
re								
os								

Notes:

Date:			Day:			Mood:		
	🍵 Breakfast		🍝 Lunch		✗ Dinner		🛏 Bedtime	
	Time	Level	Time	Level	Time	Level	Time	Level
re								
os								

Notes:

Date:			Day:			Mood:		
	🍵 Breakfast		🍝 Lunch		✗ Dinner		🛏 Bedtime	
	Time	Level	Time	Level	Time	Level	Time	Level
re								
os								

Notes:

Date:			Day:			Mood:		
	🍵 Breakfast		🍝 Lunch		✗ Dinner		🛏 Bedtime	
	Time	Level	Time	Level	Time	Level	Time	Level
re								
os								

Notes:

Date:			Day:			Mood:		
	🍵 Breakfast		🍝 Lunch		✗ Dinner		🛏 Bedtime	
	Time	Level	Time	Level	Time	Level	Time	Level
re								
os								

Notes:

Date:			Day:			Mood:		
	🍵 Breakfast		🍝 Lunch		✗ Dinner		🛏 Bedtime	
	Time	Level	Time	Level	Time	Level	Time	Level
re								
os								

Notes:

Date:			Day:			Mood:		
	☕ Breakfast		🍲 Lunch		✗ Dinner		🛏 Bedtime	
	Time	Level	Time	Level	Time	Level	Time	Level
Pre								
Pos								
Notes:								

Date:			Day:			Mood:		
	☕ Breakfast		🍲 Lunch		✗ Dinner		🛏 Bedtime	
	Time	Level	Time	Level	Time	Level	Time	Level
Pre								
Pos								
Notes:								

Date:			Day:			Mood:		
	☕ Breakfast		🍲 Lunch		✗ Dinner		🛏 Bedtime	
	Time	Level	Time	Level	Time	Level	Time	Level
Pre								
Pos								
Notes:								

Date:			Day:			Mood:		
	☕ Breakfast		🍲 Lunch		✗ Dinner		🛏 Bedtime	
	Time	Level	Time	Level	Time	Level	Time	Level
Pre								
Pos								
Notes:								

Date:			Day:			Mood:		
	☕ Breakfast		🍲 Lunch		✗ Dinner		🛏 Bedtime	
	Time	Level	Time	Level	Time	Level	Time	Level
Pre								
Pos								
Notes:								

Date:			Day:			Mood:		
	☕ Breakfast		🍲 Lunch		✗ Dinner		🛏 Bedtime	
	Time	Level	Time	Level	Time	Level	Time	Level
Pre								
Pos								
Notes:								

Date:		Day:			Mood:		
	☕ Breakfast		🍲 Lunch		✗ Dinner		🛏 Bedtime
	Time	Level	Time	Level	Time	Level	Time	Level
re								
os								

Notes:

Date:		Day:			Mood:		
	☕ Breakfast		🍲 Lunch		✗ Dinner		🛏 Bedtime
	Time	Level	Time	Level	Time	Level	Time	Level
re								
os								

Notes:

Date:		Day:			Mood:		
	☕ Breakfast		🍲 Lunch		✗ Dinner		🛏 Bedtime
	Time	Level	Time	Level	Time	Level	Time	Level
re								
os								

Notes:

Date:		Day:			Mood:		
	☕ Breakfast		🍲 Lunch		✗ Dinner		🛏 Bedtime
	Time	Level	Time	Level	Time	Level	Time	Level
re								
os								

Notes:

Date:		Day:			Mood:		
	☕ Breakfast		🍲 Lunch		✗ Dinner		🛏 Bedtime
	Time	Level	Time	Level	Time	Level	Time	Level
re								
os								

Notes:

Date:		Day:			Mood:		
	☕ Breakfast		🍲 Lunch		✗ Dinner		🛏 Bedtime
	Time	Level	Time	Level	Time	Level	Time	Level
re								
os								

Notes:

Date:			Day:			Mood:		
	☕ Breakfast		🍲 Lunch		✗ Dinner		🛏 Bedtime	
	Time	Level	Time	Level	Time	Level	Time	Level
Pre								
Pos								

Notes:

Date:			Day:			Mood:		
	☕ Breakfast		🍲 Lunch		✗ Dinner		🛏 Bedtime	
	Time	Level	Time	Level	Time	Level	Time	Level
Pre								
Pos								

Notes:

Date:			Day:			Mood:		
	☕ Breakfast		🍲 Lunch		✗ Dinner		🛏 Bedtime	
	Time	Level	Time	Level	Time	Level	Time	Level
Pre								
Pos								

Notes:

Date:			Day:			Mood:		
	☕ Breakfast		🍲 Lunch		✗ Dinner		🛏 Bedtime	
	Time	Level	Time	Level	Time	Level	Time	Level
Pre								
Pos								

Notes:

Date:			Day:			Mood:		
	☕ Breakfast		🍲 Lunch		✗ Dinner		🛏 Bedtime	
	Time	Level	Time	Level	Time	Level	Time	Level
Pre								
Pos								

Notes:

Date:			Day:			Mood:		
	☕ Breakfast		🍲 Lunch		✗ Dinner		🛏 Bedtime	
	Time	Level	Time	Level	Time	Level	Time	Level
Pre								
Pos								

Notes:

Date:			Day:			Mood:		
	☕ Breakfast		🍴 Lunch		✗ Dinner		🛏 Bedtime	
	Time	Level	Time	Level	Time	Level	Time	Level
re								
os								
otes:								

Date:			Day:			Mood:		
	☕ Breakfast		🍴 Lunch		✗ Dinner		🛏 Bedtime	
	Time	Level	Time	Level	Time	Level	Time	Level
re								
os								
otes:								

Date:			Day:			Mood:		
	☕ Breakfast		🍴 Lunch		✗ Dinner		🛏 Bedtime	
	Time	Level	Time	Level	Time	Level	Time	Level
re								
os								
otes:								

Date:			Day:			Mood:		
	☕ Breakfast		🍴 Lunch		✗ Dinner		🛏 Bedtime	
	Time	Level	Time	Level	Time	Level	Time	Level
re								
os								
otes:								

Date:			Day:			Mood:		
	☕ Breakfast		🍴 Lunch		✗ Dinner		🛏 Bedtime	
	Time	Level	Time	Level	Time	Level	Time	Level
re								
os								
otes:								

Date:			Day:			Mood:		
	☕ Breakfast		🍴 Lunch		✗ Dinner		🛏 Bedtime	
	Time	Level	Time	Level	Time	Level	Time	Level
re								
os								
otes:								

Date:			Day:			Mood:		
	☕ Breakfast		🍲 Lunch		✗ Dinner		🛏 Bedtime	
	Time	Level	Time	Level	Time	Level	Time	Level
Pre								
Pos								
Notes:								

Date:			Day:			Mood:		
	☕ Breakfast		🍲 Lunch		✗ Dinner		🛏 Bedtime	
	Time	Level	Time	Level	Time	Level	Time	Level
Pre								
Pos								
Notes:								

Date:			Day:			Mood:		
	☕ Breakfast		🍲 Lunch		✗ Dinner		🛏 Bedtime	
	Time	Level	Time	Level	Time	Level	Time	Level
Pre								
Pos								
Notes:								

Date:			Day:			Mood:		
	☕ Breakfast		🍲 Lunch		✗ Dinner		🛏 Bedtime	
	Time	Level	Time	Level	Time	Level	Time	Level
Pre								
Pos								
Notes:								

Date:			Day:			Mood:		
	☕ Breakfast		🍲 Lunch		✗ Dinner		🛏 Bedtime	
	Time	Level	Time	Level	Time	Level	Time	Level
Pre								
Pos								
Notes:								

Date:			Day:			Mood:		
	☕ Breakfast		🍲 Lunch		✗ Dinner		🛏 Bedtime	
	Time	Level	Time	Level	Time	Level	Time	Level
Pre								
Pos								
Notes:								

Date:		Day:			Mood:		
	🍵 Breakfast		🍔 Lunch		✗ Dinner		🛏 Bedtime
	Time	Level	Time	Level	Time	Level	Time	Level
re								
os								

Notes:

Date:		Day:			Mood:		
	🍵 Breakfast		🍔 Lunch		✗ Dinner		🛏 Bedtime
	Time	Level	Time	Level	Time	Level	Time	Level
re								
os								

Notes:

Date:		Day:			Mood:		
	🍵 Breakfast		🍔 Lunch		✗ Dinner		🛏 Bedtime
	Time	Level	Time	Level	Time	Level	Time	Level
re								
os								

Notes:

Date:		Day:			Mood:		
	🍵 Breakfast		🍔 Lunch		✗ Dinner		🛏 Bedtime
	Time	Level	Time	Level	Time	Level	Time	Level
re								
os								

Notes:

Date:		Day:			Mood:		
	🍵 Breakfast		🍔 Lunch		✗ Dinner		🛏 Bedtime
	Time	Level	Time	Level	Time	Level	Time	Level
re								
os								

Notes:

Date:		Day:			Mood:		
	🍵 Breakfast		🍔 Lunch		✗ Dinner		🛏 Bedtime
	Time	Level	Time	Level	Time	Level	Time	Level
re								
os								

Notes:

Date:			Day:			Mood:		
	☕ Breakfast		🥣 Lunch		✗ Dinner		🛏 Bedtime	
	Time	Level	Time	Level	Time	Level	Time	Level
Pre								
Pos								
Notes:								

Date:			Day:			Mood:		
	☕ Breakfast		🥣 Lunch		✗ Dinner		🛏 Bedtime	
	Time	Level	Time	Level	Time	Level	Time	Level
Pre								
Pos								
Notes:								

Date:			Day:			Mood:		
	☕ Breakfast		🥣 Lunch		✗ Dinner		🛏 Bedtime	
	Time	Level	Time	Level	Time	Level	Time	Level
Pre								
Pos								
Notes:								

Date:			Day:			Mood:		
	☕ Breakfast		🥣 Lunch		✗ Dinner		🛏 Bedtime	
	Time	Level	Time	Level	Time	Level	Time	Level
Pre								
Pos								
Notes:								

Date:			Day:			Mood:		
	☕ Breakfast		🥣 Lunch		✗ Dinner		🛏 Bedtime	
	Time	Level	Time	Level	Time	Level	Time	Level
Pre								
Pos								
Notes:								

Date:			Day:			Mood:		
	☕ Breakfast		🥣 Lunch		✗ Dinner		🛏 Bedtime	
	Time	Level	Time	Level	Time	Level	Time	Level
Pre								
Pos								
Notes:								

Date: _____ **Day:** _____ **Mood:** _____

	☕ Breakfast		🍽 Lunch		✗ Dinner		🛏 Bedtime	
	Time	Level	Time	Level	Time	Level	Time	Level
re								
os								

Notes:

Date: _____ **Day:** _____ **Mood:** _____

	☕ Breakfast		🍽 Lunch		✗ Dinner		🛏 Bedtime	
	Time	Level	Time	Level	Time	Level	Time	Level
re								
os								

Notes:

Date: _____ **Day:** _____ **Mood:** _____

	☕ Breakfast		🍽 Lunch		✗ Dinner		🛏 Bedtime	
	Time	Level	Time	Level	Time	Level	Time	Level
re								
os								

Notes:

Date: _____ **Day:** _____ **Mood:** _____

	☕ Breakfast		🍽 Lunch		✗ Dinner		🛏 Bedtime	
	Time	Level	Time	Level	Time	Level	Time	Level
re								
os								

Notes:

Date: _____ **Day:** _____ **Mood:** _____

	☕ Breakfast		🍽 Lunch		✗ Dinner		🛏 Bedtime	
	Time	Level	Time	Level	Time	Level	Time	Level
re								
os								

Notes:

Date: _____ **Day:** _____ **Mood:** _____

	☕ Breakfast		🍽 Lunch		✗ Dinner		🛏 Bedtime	
	Time	Level	Time	Level	Time	Level	Time	Level
re								
os								

Notes:

Date:		Day:			Mood:		
	☕ Breakfast		🍽 Lunch		✗ Dinner		🛏 Bedtime
	Time	Level	Time	Level	Time	Level	Time	Level
Pre								
Pos								

Notes:

Date:		Day:			Mood:		
	☕ Breakfast		🍽 Lunch		✗ Dinner		🛏 Bedtime
	Time	Level	Time	Level	Time	Level	Time	Level
Pre								
Pos								

Notes:

Date:		Day:			Mood:		
	☕ Breakfast		🍽 Lunch		✗ Dinner		🛏 Bedtime
	Time	Level	Time	Level	Time	Level	Time	Level
Pre								
Pos								

Notes:

Date:		Day:			Mood:		
	☕ Breakfast		🍽 Lunch		✗ Dinner		🛏 Bedtime
	Time	Level	Time	Level	Time	Level	Time	Level
Pre								
Pos								

Notes:

Date:		Day:			Mood:		
	☕ Breakfast		🍽 Lunch		✗ Dinner		🛏 Bedtime
	Time	Level	Time	Level	Time	Level	Time	Level
Pre								
Pos								

Notes:

Date:		Day:			Mood:		
	☕ Breakfast		🍽 Lunch		✗ Dinner		🛏 Bedtime
	Time	Level	Time	Level	Time	Level	Time	Level
Pre								
Pos								

Notes:

Date:			Day:			Mood:		
	🍵 Breakfast		🍔 Lunch		✗ Dinner		🛏 Bedtime	
	Time	Level	Time	Level	Time	Level	Time	Level
re								
os								

Notes:

Date:			Day:			Mood:		
	🍵 Breakfast		🍔 Lunch		✗ Dinner		🛏 Bedtime	
	Time	Level	Time	Level	Time	Level	Time	Level
re								
os								

Notes:

Date:			Day:			Mood:		
	🍵 Breakfast		🍔 Lunch		✗ Dinner		🛏 Bedtime	
	Time	Level	Time	Level	Time	Level	Time	Level
re								
os								

Notes:

Date:			Day:			Mood:		
	🍵 Breakfast		🍔 Lunch		✗ Dinner		🛏 Bedtime	
	Time	Level	Time	Level	Time	Level	Time	Level
re								
os								

Notes:

Date:			Day:			Mood:		
	🍵 Breakfast		🍔 Lunch		✗ Dinner		🛏 Bedtime	
	Time	Level	Time	Level	Time	Level	Time	Level
re								
os								

Notes:

Date:			Day:			Mood:		
	🍵 Breakfast		🍔 Lunch		✗ Dinner		🛏 Bedtime	
	Time	Level	Time	Level	Time	Level	Time	Level
re								
os								

Notes:

Date:			Day:			Mood:		
	☕ Breakfast		🍜 Lunch		✗ Dinner		🛏 Bedtime	
	Time	Level	Time	Level	Time	Level	Time	Level
Pre								
Pos								
Notes:								

Date:			Day:			Mood:		
	☕ Breakfast		🍜 Lunch		✗ Dinner		🛏 Bedtime	
	Time	Level	Time	Level	Time	Level	Time	Level
Pre								
Pos								
Notes:								

Date:			Day:			Mood:		
	☕ Breakfast		🍜 Lunch		✗ Dinner		🛏 Bedtime	
	Time	Level	Time	Level	Time	Level	Time	Level
Pre								
Pos								
Notes:								

Date:			Day:			Mood:		
	☕ Breakfast		🍜 Lunch		✗ Dinner		🛏 Bedtime	
	Time	Level	Time	Level	Time	Level	Time	Level
Pre								
Pos								
Notes:								

Date:			Day:			Mood:		
	☕ Breakfast		🍜 Lunch		✗ Dinner		🛏 Bedtime	
	Time	Level	Time	Level	Time	Level	Time	Level
Pre								
Pos								
Notes:								

Date:			Day:			Mood:		
	☕ Breakfast		🍜 Lunch		✗ Dinner		🛏 Bedtime	
	Time	Level	Time	Level	Time	Level	Time	Level
Pre								
Pos								
Notes:								

Date:			Day:			Mood:		
	🍵 Breakfast		🍔 Lunch		✗ Dinner		🛏 Bedtime	
	Time	Level	Time	Level	Time	Level	Time	Level
re								
os								

Notes:

Date:			Day:			Mood:		
	🍵 Breakfast		🍔 Lunch		✗ Dinner		🛏 Bedtime	
	Time	Level	Time	Level	Time	Level	Time	Level
re								
os								

Notes:

Date:			Day:			Mood:		
	🍵 Breakfast		🍔 Lunch		✗ Dinner		🛏 Bedtime	
	Time	Level	Time	Level	Time	Level	Time	Level
re								
os								

Notes:

Date:			Day:			Mood:		
	🍵 Breakfast		🍔 Lunch		✗ Dinner		🛏 Bedtime	
	Time	Level	Time	Level	Time	Level	Time	Level
re								
os								

Notes:

Date:			Day:			Mood:		
	🍵 Breakfast		🍔 Lunch		✗ Dinner		🛏 Bedtime	
	Time	Level	Time	Level	Time	Level	Time	Level
re								
os								

Notes:

Date:			Day:			Mood:		
	🍵 Breakfast		🍔 Lunch		✗ Dinner		🛏 Bedtime	
	Time	Level	Time	Level	Time	Level	Time	Level
re								
os								

Notes:

Date:			Day:			Mood:		
	☕ Breakfast		🍲 Lunch		✕ Dinner		🛏 Bedtime	
	Time	Level	Time	Level	Time	Level	Time	Level
Pre								
Pos								
Notes:								

Date:			Day:			Mood:		
	☕ Breakfast		🍲 Lunch		✕ Dinner		🛏 Bedtime	
	Time	Level	Time	Level	Time	Level	Time	Level
Pre								
Pos								
Notes:								

Date:			Day:			Mood:		
	☕ Breakfast		🍲 Lunch		✕ Dinner		🛏 Bedtime	
	Time	Level	Time	Level	Time	Level	Time	Level
Pre								
Pos								
Notes:								

Date:			Day:			Mood:		
	☕ Breakfast		🍲 Lunch		✕ Dinner		🛏 Bedtime	
	Time	Level	Time	Level	Time	Level	Time	Level
Pre								
Pos								
Notes:								

Date:			Day:			Mood:		
	☕ Breakfast		🍲 Lunch		✕ Dinner		🛏 Bedtime	
	Time	Level	Time	Level	Time	Level	Time	Level
Pre								
Pos								
Notes:								

Date:			Day:			Mood:		
	☕ Breakfast		🍲 Lunch		✕ Dinner		🛏 Bedtime	
	Time	Level	Time	Level	Time	Level	Time	Level
Pre								
Pos								
Notes:								

Date:			Day:			Mood:		
	☕ Breakfast		🍔 Lunch		✕ Dinner		🛏 Bedtime	
	Time	Level	Time	Level	Time	Level	Time	Level
re								
os								

Notes:

Date:			Day:			Mood:		
	☕ Breakfast		🍔 Lunch		✕ Dinner		🛏 Bedtime	
	Time	Level	Time	Level	Time	Level	Time	Level
re								
os								

Notes:

Date:			Day:			Mood:		
	☕ Breakfast		🍔 Lunch		✕ Dinner		🛏 Bedtime	
	Time	Level	Time	Level	Time	Level	Time	Level
re								
os								

Notes:

Date:			Day:			Mood:		
	☕ Breakfast		🍔 Lunch		✕ Dinner		🛏 Bedtime	
	Time	Level	Time	Level	Time	Level	Time	Level
re								
os								

Notes:

Date:			Day:			Mood:		
	☕ Breakfast		🍔 Lunch		✕ Dinner		🛏 Bedtime	
	Time	Level	Time	Level	Time	Level	Time	Level
re								
os								

Notes:

Date:			Day:			Mood:		
	☕ Breakfast		🍔 Lunch		✕ Dinner		🛏 Bedtime	
	Time	Level	Time	Level	Time	Level	Time	Level
re								
os								

Notes:

Date:			Day:			Mood:		
	☕ Breakfast		🍴 Lunch		✗ Dinner		🛏 Bedtime	
	Time	Level	Time	Level	Time	Level	Time	Level
Pre								
Pos								

Notes:

Date:			Day:			Mood:		
	☕ Breakfast		🍴 Lunch		✗ Dinner		🛏 Bedtime	
	Time	Level	Time	Level	Time	Level	Time	Level
Pre								
Pos								

Notes:

Date:			Day:			Mood:		
	☕ Breakfast		🍴 Lunch		✗ Dinner		🛏 Bedtime	
	Time	Level	Time	Level	Time	Level	Time	Level
Pre								
Pos								

Notes:

Date:			Day:			Mood:		
	☕ Breakfast		🍴 Lunch		✗ Dinner		🛏 Bedtime	
	Time	Level	Time	Level	Time	Level	Time	Level
Pre								
Pos								

Notes:

Date:			Day:			Mood:		
	☕ Breakfast		🍴 Lunch		✗ Dinner		🛏 Bedtime	
	Time	Level	Time	Level	Time	Level	Time	Level
Pre								
Pos								

Notes:

Date:			Day:			Mood:		
	☕ Breakfast		🍴 Lunch		✗ Dinner		🛏 Bedtime	
	Time	Level	Time	Level	Time	Level	Time	Level
Pre								
Pos								

Notes:

Date:			Day:			Mood:				
	☕ **Breakfast**		🍴 **Lunch**		✕ **Dinner**		🛏 **Bedtime**		
	Time	Level	Time	Level	Time	Level	Time	Level
re								
os								

Notes:

Date:			Day:			Mood:				
	☕ **Breakfast**		🍴 **Lunch**		✕ **Dinner**		🛏 **Bedtime**		
	Time	Level	Time	Level	Time	Level	Time	Level
re								
os								

Notes:

Date:			Day:			Mood:				
	☕ **Breakfast**		🍴 **Lunch**		✕ **Dinner**		🛏 **Bedtime**		
	Time	Level	Time	Level	Time	Level	Time	Level
re								
os								

Notes:

Date:			Day:			Mood:				
	☕ **Breakfast**		🍴 **Lunch**		✕ **Dinner**		🛏 **Bedtime**		
	Time	Level	Time	Level	Time	Level	Time	Level
re								
os								

Notes:

Date:			Day:			Mood:				
	☕ **Breakfast**		🍴 **Lunch**		✕ **Dinner**		🛏 **Bedtime**		
	Time	Level	Time	Level	Time	Level	Time	Level
re								
os								

Notes:

Date:			Day:			Mood:				
	☕ **Breakfast**		🍴 **Lunch**		✕ **Dinner**		🛏 **Bedtime**		
	Time	Level	Time	Level	Time	Level	Time	Level
re								
os								

Notes:

Date:		Day:			Mood:		
	🍵 Breakfast		🍚 Lunch		✗ Dinner		🛏 Bedtime
	Time	Level	Time	Level	Time	Level	Time	Level
Pre								
Pos								

Notes:

Date:		Day:			Mood:		
	🍵 Breakfast		🍚 Lunch		✗ Dinner		🛏 Bedtime
	Time	Level	Time	Level	Time	Level	Time	Level
Pre								
Pos								

Notes:

Date:		Day:			Mood:		
	🍵 Breakfast		🍚 Lunch		✗ Dinner		🛏 Bedtime
	Time	Level	Time	Level	Time	Level	Time	Level
Pre								
Pos								

Notes:

Date:		Day:			Mood:		
	🍵 Breakfast		🍚 Lunch		✗ Dinner		🛏 Bedtime
	Time	Level	Time	Level	Time	Level	Time	Level
Pre								
Pos								

Notes:

Date:		Day:			Mood:		
	🍵 Breakfast		🍚 Lunch		✗ Dinner		🛏 Bedtime
	Time	Level	Time	Level	Time	Level	Time	Level
Pre								
Pos								

Notes:

Date:		Day:			Mood:		
	🍵 Breakfast		🍚 Lunch		✗ Dinner		🛏 Bedtime
	Time	Level	Time	Level	Time	Level	Time	Level
Pre								
Pos								

Notes:

Date:			Day:			Mood:		
	☕ Breakfast		🍲 Lunch		✗ Dinner		🛏 Bedtime	
	Time	Level	Time	Level	Time	Level	Time	Level
re								
os								

Notes:

Date:			Day:			Mood:		
	☕ Breakfast		🍲 Lunch		✗ Dinner		🛏 Bedtime	
	Time	Level	Time	Level	Time	Level	Time	Level
re								
os								

Notes:

Date:			Day:			Mood:		
	☕ Breakfast		🍲 Lunch		✗ Dinner		🛏 Bedtime	
	Time	Level	Time	Level	Time	Level	Time	Level
re								
os								

Notes:

Date:			Day:			Mood:		
	☕ Breakfast		🍲 Lunch		✗ Dinner		🛏 Bedtime	
	Time	Level	Time	Level	Time	Level	Time	Level
re								
os								

Notes:

Date:			Day:			Mood:		
	☕ Breakfast		🍲 Lunch		✗ Dinner		🛏 Bedtime	
	Time	Level	Time	Level	Time	Level	Time	Level
re								
os								

Notes:

Date:			Day:			Mood:		
	☕ Breakfast		🍲 Lunch		✗ Dinner		🛏 Bedtime	
	Time	Level	Time	Level	Time	Level	Time	Level
re								
os								

Notes:

Date:			Day:			Mood:		
	☕ Breakfast		🍴 Lunch		✕ Dinner		🛏 Bedtime	
	Time	Level	Time	Level	Time	Level	Time	Level
Pre								
Pos								
Notes:								

Date:			Day:			Mood:		
	☕ Breakfast		🍴 Lunch		✕ Dinner		🛏 Bedtime	
	Time	Level	Time	Level	Time	Level	Time	Level
Pre								
Pos								
Notes:								

Date:			Day:			Mood:		
	☕ Breakfast		🍴 Lunch		✕ Dinner		🛏 Bedtime	
	Time	Level	Time	Level	Time	Level	Time	Level
Pre								
Pos								
Notes:								

Date:			Day:			Mood:		
	☕ Breakfast		🍴 Lunch		✕ Dinner		🛏 Bedtime	
	Time	Level	Time	Level	Time	Level	Time	Level
Pre								
Pos								
Notes:								

Date:			Day:			Mood:		
	☕ Breakfast		🍴 Lunch		✕ Dinner		🛏 Bedtime	
	Time	Level	Time	Level	Time	Level	Time	Level
Pre								
Pos								
Notes:								

Date:			Day:			Mood:		
	☕ Breakfast		🍴 Lunch		✕ Dinner		🛏 Bedtime	
	Time	Level	Time	Level	Time	Level	Time	Level
Pre								
Pos								
Notes:								

Date:			Day:			Mood:		
	☕ Breakfast		🍴 Lunch		✗ Dinner		🛏 Bedtime	
	Time	Level	Time	Level	Time	Level	Time	Level
re								
os								
otes:								

Date:			Day:			Mood:		
	☕ Breakfast		🍴 Lunch		✗ Dinner		🛏 Bedtime	
	Time	Level	Time	Level	Time	Level	Time	Level
re								
os								
otes:								

Date:			Day:			Mood:		
	☕ Breakfast		🍴 Lunch		✗ Dinner		🛏 Bedtime	
	Time	Level	Time	Level	Time	Level	Time	Level
re								
os								
otes:								

Date:			Day:			Mood:		
	☕ Breakfast		🍴 Lunch		✗ Dinner		🛏 Bedtime	
	Time	Level	Time	Level	Time	Level	Time	Level
re								
os								
otes:								

Date:			Day:			Mood:		
	☕ Breakfast		🍴 Lunch		✗ Dinner		🛏 Bedtime	
	Time	Level	Time	Level	Time	Level	Time	Level
re								
os								
otes:								

Date:			Day:			Mood:		
	☕ Breakfast		🍴 Lunch		✗ Dinner		🛏 Bedtime	
	Time	Level	Time	Level	Time	Level	Time	Level
re								
os								
otes:								

Date:		Day:		Mood:	

	☕ Breakfast		🍽 Lunch		✕ Dinner		🛏 Bedtime	
	Time	Level	Time	Level	Time	Level	Time	Level
Pre								
Pos								

Notes:

Date:		Day:		Mood:	

	☕ Breakfast		🍽 Lunch		✕ Dinner		🛏 Bedtime	
	Time	Level	Time	Level	Time	Level	Time	Level
Pre								
Pos								

Notes:

Date:		Day:		Mood:	

	☕ Breakfast		🍽 Lunch		✕ Dinner		🛏 Bedtime	
	Time	Level	Time	Level	Time	Level	Time	Level
Pre								
Pos								

Notes:

Date:		Day:		Mood:	

	☕ Breakfast		🍽 Lunch		✕ Dinner		🛏 Bedtime	
	Time	Level	Time	Level	Time	Level	Time	Level
Pre								
Pos								

Notes:

Date:		Day:		Mood:	

	☕ Breakfast		🍽 Lunch		✕ Dinner		🛏 Bedtime	
	Time	Level	Time	Level	Time	Level	Time	Level
Pre								
Pos								

Notes:

Date:		Day:		Mood:	

	☕ Breakfast		🍽 Lunch		✕ Dinner		🛏 Bedtime	
	Time	Level	Time	Level	Time	Level	Time	Level
Pre								
Pos								

Notes:

Date:		Day:			Mood:		
☕ Breakfast		🍲 Lunch		✗ Dinner		🛏 Bedtime	
Time	Level	Time	Level	Time	Level	Time	Level
re							
os							

otes:

Date:		Day:			Mood:		
☕ Breakfast		🍲 Lunch		✗ Dinner		🛏 Bedtime	
Time	Level	Time	Level	Time	Level	Time	Level
re							
os							

otes:

Date:		Day:			Mood:		
☕ Breakfast		🍲 Lunch		✗ Dinner		🛏 Bedtime	
Time	Level	Time	Level	Time	Level	Time	Level
re							
os							

otes:

Date:		Day:			Mood:		
☕ Breakfast		🍲 Lunch		✗ Dinner		🛏 Bedtime	
Time	Level	Time	Level	Time	Level	Time	Level
re							
os							

otes:

Date:		Day:			Mood:		
☕ Breakfast		🍲 Lunch		✗ Dinner		🛏 Bedtime	
Time	Level	Time	Level	Time	Level	Time	Level
re							
os							

otes:

Date:		Day:			Mood:		
☕ Breakfast		🍲 Lunch		✗ Dinner		🛏 Bedtime	
Time	Level	Time	Level	Time	Level	Time	Level
re							
os							

otes:

Date:			Day:			Mood:		
	☕ Breakfast		🍲 Lunch		✕ Dinner		🛏 Bedtime	
	Time	Level	Time	Level	Time	Level	Time	Level
Pre								
Pos								

Notes:

Date:			Day:			Mood:		
	☕ Breakfast		🍲 Lunch		✕ Dinner		🛏 Bedtime	
	Time	Level	Time	Level	Time	Level	Time	Level
Pre								
Pos								

Notes:

Date:			Day:			Mood:		
	☕ Breakfast		🍲 Lunch		✕ Dinner		🛏 Bedtime	
	Time	Level	Time	Level	Time	Level	Time	Level
Pre								
Pos								

Notes:

Date:			Day:			Mood:		
	☕ Breakfast		🍲 Lunch		✕ Dinner		🛏 Bedtime	
	Time	Level	Time	Level	Time	Level	Time	Level
Pre								
Pos								

Notes:

Date:			Day:			Mood:		
	☕ Breakfast		🍲 Lunch		✕ Dinner		🛏 Bedtime	
	Time	Level	Time	Level	Time	Level	Time	Level
Pre								
Pos								

Notes:

Date:			Day:			Mood:		
	☕ Breakfast		🍲 Lunch		✕ Dinner		🛏 Bedtime	
	Time	Level	Time	Level	Time	Level	Time	Level
Pre								
Pos								

Notes:

Date:			Day:			Mood:		
	☕ Breakfast		🍔 Lunch		✗ Dinner		🛏 Bedtime	
	Time	Level	Time	Level	Time	Level	Time	Level
re								
os								

Notes:

Date:			Day:			Mood:		
	☕ Breakfast		🍔 Lunch		✗ Dinner		🛏 Bedtime	
	Time	Level	Time	Level	Time	Level	Time	Level
re								
os								

Notes:

Date:			Day:			Mood:		
	☕ Breakfast		🍔 Lunch		✗ Dinner		🛏 Bedtime	
	Time	Level	Time	Level	Time	Level	Time	Level
re								
os								

Notes:

Date:			Day:			Mood:		
	☕ Breakfast		🍔 Lunch		✗ Dinner		🛏 Bedtime	
	Time	Level	Time	Level	Time	Level	Time	Level
re								
os								

Notes:

Date:			Day:			Mood:		
	☕ Breakfast		🍔 Lunch		✗ Dinner		🛏 Bedtime	
	Time	Level	Time	Level	Time	Level	Time	Level
re								
os								

Notes:

Date:			Day:			Mood:		
	☕ Breakfast		🍔 Lunch		✗ Dinner		🛏 Bedtime	
	Time	Level	Time	Level	Time	Level	Time	Level
re								
os								

Notes:

Date:			Day:			Mood:		
	🍵 Breakfast		🍲 Lunch		✗ Dinner		🛏 Bedtime	
	Time	Level	Time	Level	Time	Level	Time	Level
Pre								
Pos								
Notes:								

Date:			Day:			Mood:		
	🍵 Breakfast		🍲 Lunch		✗ Dinner		🛏 Bedtime	
	Time	Level	Time	Level	Time	Level	Time	Level
Pre								
Pos								
Notes:								

Date:			Day:			Mood:		
	🍵 Breakfast		🍲 Lunch		✗ Dinner		🛏 Bedtime	
	Time	Level	Time	Level	Time	Level	Time	Level
Pre								
Pos								
Notes:								

Date:			Day:			Mood:		
	🍵 Breakfast		🍲 Lunch		✗ Dinner		🛏 Bedtime	
	Time	Level	Time	Level	Time	Level	Time	Level
Pre								
Pos								
Notes:								

Date:			Day:			Mood:		
	🍵 Breakfast		🍲 Lunch		✗ Dinner		🛏 Bedtime	
	Time	Level	Time	Level	Time	Level	Time	Level
Pre								
Pos								
Notes:								

Date:			Day:			Mood:		
	🍵 Breakfast		🍲 Lunch		✗ Dinner		🛏 Bedtime	
	Time	Level	Time	Level	Time	Level	Time	Level
Pre								
Pos								
Notes:								

Date:			Day:			Mood:		
	🍵 Breakfast		🍔 Lunch		✗ Dinner		🛏 Bedtime	
	Time	Level	Time	Level	Time	Level	Time	Level
re								
os								

Notes:

Date:			Day:			Mood:		
	🍵 Breakfast		🍔 Lunch		✗ Dinner		🛏 Bedtime	
	Time	Level	Time	Level	Time	Level	Time	Level
re								
os								

Notes:

Date:			Day:			Mood:		
	🍵 Breakfast		🍔 Lunch		✗ Dinner		🛏 Bedtime	
	Time	Level	Time	Level	Time	Level	Time	Level
re								
os								

Notes:

Date:			Day:			Mood:		
	🍵 Breakfast		🍔 Lunch		✗ Dinner		🛏 Bedtime	
	Time	Level	Time	Level	Time	Level	Time	Level
re								
os								

Notes:

Date:			Day:			Mood:		
	🍵 Breakfast		🍔 Lunch		✗ Dinner		🛏 Bedtime	
	Time	Level	Time	Level	Time	Level	Time	Level
re								
os								

Notes:

Date:			Day:			Mood:		
	🍵 Breakfast		🍔 Lunch		✗ Dinner		🛏 Bedtime	
	Time	Level	Time	Level	Time	Level	Time	Level
re								
os								

Notes:

Date:			Day:			Mood:		
	☕ Breakfast		🍴 Lunch		✗ Dinner		🛏 Bedtime	
	Time	Level	Time	Level	Time	Level	Time	Level
Pre								
Pos								
Notes:								

Date:			Day:			Mood:		
	☕ Breakfast		🍴 Lunch		✗ Dinner		🛏 Bedtime	
	Time	Level	Time	Level	Time	Level	Time	Level
Pre								
Pos								
Notes:								

Date:			Day:			Mood:		
	☕ Breakfast		🍴 Lunch		✗ Dinner		🛏 Bedtime	
	Time	Level	Time	Level	Time	Level	Time	Level
Pre								
Pos								
Notes:								

Date:			Day:			Mood:		
	☕ Breakfast		🍴 Lunch		✗ Dinner		🛏 Bedtime	
	Time	Level	Time	Level	Time	Level	Time	Level
Pre								
Pos								
Notes:								

Date:			Day:			Mood:		
	☕ Breakfast		🍴 Lunch		✗ Dinner		🛏 Bedtime	
	Time	Level	Time	Level	Time	Level	Time	Level
Pre								
Pos								
Notes:								

Date:			Day:			Mood:		
	☕ Breakfast		🍴 Lunch		✗ Dinner		🛏 Bedtime	
	Time	Level	Time	Level	Time	Level	Time	Level
Pre								
Pos								
Notes:								

Date:			Day:			Mood:		
	☕ Breakfast		🍝 Lunch		✗ Dinner		🛏 Bedtime	
	Time	Level	Time	Level	Time	Level	Time	Level
re								
os								

Notes:

Date:			Day:			Mood:		
	☕ Breakfast		🍝 Lunch		✗ Dinner		🛏 Bedtime	
	Time	Level	Time	Level	Time	Level	Time	Level
re								
os								

Notes:

Date:			Day:			Mood:		
	☕ Breakfast		🍝 Lunch		✗ Dinner		🛏 Bedtime	
	Time	Level	Time	Level	Time	Level	Time	Level
re								
os								

Notes:

Date:			Day:			Mood:		
	☕ Breakfast		🍝 Lunch		✗ Dinner		🛏 Bedtime	
	Time	Level	Time	Level	Time	Level	Time	Level
re								
os								

Notes:

Date:			Day:			Mood:		
	☕ Breakfast		🍝 Lunch		✗ Dinner		🛏 Bedtime	
	Time	Level	Time	Level	Time	Level	Time	Level
re								
os								

Notes:

Date:			Day:			Mood:		
	☕ Breakfast		🍝 Lunch		✗ Dinner		🛏 Bedtime	
	Time	Level	Time	Level	Time	Level	Time	Level
re								
os								

Notes:

Date:			Day:			Mood:		
	☕ Breakfast		🍽 Lunch		✕ Dinner		🛏 Bedtime	
	Time	Level	Time	Level	Time	Level	Time	Level
Pre								
Pos								
Notes:								

Date:			Day:			Mood:		
	☕ Breakfast		🍽 Lunch		✕ Dinner		🛏 Bedtime	
	Time	Level	Time	Level	Time	Level	Time	Level
Pre								
Pos								
Notes:								

Date:			Day:			Mood:		
	☕ Breakfast		🍽 Lunch		✕ Dinner		🛏 Bedtime	
	Time	Level	Time	Level	Time	Level	Time	Level
Pre								
Pos								
Notes:								

Date:			Day:			Mood:		
	☕ Breakfast		🍽 Lunch		✕ Dinner		🛏 Bedtime	
	Time	Level	Time	Level	Time	Level	Time	Level
Pre								
Pos								
Notes:								

Date:			Day:			Mood:		
	☕ Breakfast		🍽 Lunch		✕ Dinner		🛏 Bedtime	
	Time	Level	Time	Level	Time	Level	Time	Level
Pre								
Pos								
Notes:								

Date:			Day:			Mood:		
	☕ Breakfast		🍽 Lunch		✕ Dinner		🛏 Bedtime	
	Time	Level	Time	Level	Time	Level	Time	Level
Pre								
Pos								
Notes:								

Date:			Day:			Mood:		
	☕ Breakfast		🍴 Lunch		✗ Dinner		🛏 Bedtime	
	Time	Level	Time	Level	Time	Level	Time	Level
re								
os								

Notes:

Date:			Day:			Mood:		
	☕ Breakfast		🍴 Lunch		✗ Dinner		🛏 Bedtime	
	Time	Level	Time	Level	Time	Level	Time	Level
re								
os								

Notes:

Date:			Day:			Mood:		
	☕ Breakfast		🍴 Lunch		✗ Dinner		🛏 Bedtime	
	Time	Level	Time	Level	Time	Level	Time	Level
re								
os								

Notes:

Date:			Day:			Mood:		
	☕ Breakfast		🍴 Lunch		✗ Dinner		🛏 Bedtime	
	Time	Level	Time	Level	Time	Level	Time	Level
re								
os								

Notes:

Date:			Day:			Mood:		
	☕ Breakfast		🍴 Lunch		✗ Dinner		🛏 Bedtime	
	Time	Level	Time	Level	Time	Level	Time	Level
re								
os								

Notes:

Date:			Day:			Mood:		
	☕ Breakfast		🍴 Lunch		✗ Dinner		🛏 Bedtime	
	Time	Level	Time	Level	Time	Level	Time	Level
re								
os								

Notes:

Made in the USA
Middletown, DE
24 June 2022